近红外多功能纳米探针的构建
及其在胃肠道恶性肿瘤诊断与治疗中的应用

杨正阳 / 著

东南大学出版社
·南京·

内容提要

本书首先介绍了胃肠道恶性肿瘤的流行病学背景和早期诊断的重要性。随后,详细阐述了近红外多功能纳米探针的设计与构建过程,包括其在靶向性、成像能力和药物递送方面的优势。重点介绍了纳米探针在胃肠道恶性肿瘤诊断中的应用,如通过近红外荧光成像和光声成像技术实现对肿瘤的高灵敏度和高特异性检测。此外,还探讨了纳米探针在治疗中的应用,包括光动力治疗和光热治疗等方法,这些方法能够有效杀伤肿瘤细胞,同时减少对正常组织的损伤。最后讨论了纳米探针在临床应用中的潜在挑战和未来发展方向,强调了进一步优化纳米探针的生物相容性和稳定性的重要性。

图书在版编目(CIP)数据

近红外多功能纳米探针的构建及其在胃肠道恶性肿瘤诊断与治疗中的应用 / 杨正阳著. -- 南京:东南大学出版社,2025.4. -- ISBN 978-7-5766-2047-4

Ⅰ. R735

中国国家版本馆 CIP 数据核字第 20259934QG 号

近红外多功能纳米探针的构建及其在胃肠道恶性肿瘤诊断与治疗中的应用

Jinhongwai Duogongneng Nami Tanzhen De Goujian Jiqi Zai Weichangdao Exing Zhongliu Zhenduan Yu Zhiliao Zhong De Yingyong

著 者	杨正阳
责任编辑	张 烨　　责任校对　子雪莲　　封面设计　王 玥　　责任印制　周荣虎
出版发行	东南大学出版社
出 版 人	白云飞
社　　址	南京市四牌楼 2 号(邮编:210096　电话:025 - 83793330)
经　　销	全国各地新华书店
印　　刷	广东虎彩云印刷有限公司
开　　本	700mm×1000mm　1/16
印　　张	8.5
字　　数	167 千字
版　　次	2025 年 4 月第 1 版
印　　次	2025 年 4 月第 1 次印刷
书　　号	ISBN 978-7-5766-2047-4
定　　价	68.00 元

本社图书若有印装质量问题,请直接与营销部调换。电话(传真):025 - 83791830

前言

在当今医学领域，胃肠道恶性肿瘤无疑是一个重大的挑战，它严重威胁着人类的健康和生命，给患者及其家庭带来了巨大的痛苦和负担。然而，随着科技的不断进步，新的诊断和治疗方法正不断涌现，为战胜这一顽疾带来了新的希望。其中纳米生物这一领域越来越受到人们的关注。纳米医学可以为胃肠道恶性肿瘤的诊断与治疗提供许多潜在的好处，主要包括以下优势：① 纳米颗粒可以被生物分子功能化，使其能够靶向肿瘤组织，定位于目标病灶；② 纳米颗粒通常可以通过表面修饰，包裹或添加配方来克服普通化疗药物溶解性和稳定性的问题；③ 纳米颗粒具有新颖的物理性质，如近红外荧光成像、光声成像等，可用于生物成像；④ 纳米颗粒通常由数千个具有高表面积的物质组成，因此可以携带更高的治疗载荷，对肿瘤组织杀伤能力更强；⑤ 纳米颗粒可通过被动或主动靶向，在肿瘤部位有效累积，从而显著降低器官非特异性毒性。但是，由于不同的纳米药物具有不同的理化性质，导致其具有不同的分布特性和半衰期等。因此，如何将纳米药物应用于胃肠道恶性肿瘤的诊断与治疗，已成为一个挑战性的科学问题。

本书系统深入地阐述了近红外多功能纳米探针的构建原理、特性、优势以及在胃肠道恶性肿瘤诊断与治疗中的多元应用。从纳米材料的精心筛选与巧妙合成，到探针的精细设计与精准制备；从细胞与动物实验的严谨开展，到临床应用前景的科学展望，笔者皆以详尽而精准的笔触予以呈现，为读者勾勒出一幅完整而清晰的技术发展蓝图。书中全面介绍了近红外光独特的光学特性，如良好的组织穿透性与较低的生物组织自发荧光干扰,这些特性使其成为理想的肿瘤检测与治疗光源。而基于此构建的多功能纳米探针,巧妙融合了靶向识别、荧光成像、光热治疗、光动力治疗等多种功能于一体,实现了肿瘤的精准定位、可视化诊断以及高效联合治疗,为胃肠道恶性肿瘤的诊疗开辟了崭新的路径。

  本书在阐述理论知识的同时,紧密结合大量前沿研究成果与实际案例,深入浅出地剖析了近红外多功能纳米探针在提高肿瘤早期诊断准确率、实现肿瘤精准分期分型、优化治疗方案以及监测治疗效果等方面的显著优势与潜在价值。这不仅有助于读者深入理解相关技术的科学内涵与应用逻辑,更为从事胃肠道恶性肿瘤研究的科研人员、临床医生以及相关专业的研究生提供了丰富的灵感源泉与极具借鉴意义的实践指导。

  在当今科技飞速发展的时代,多学科交叉融合已成为推动医学进步的强大动力。本书的创作充分彰显了这一理念,有机整合了材料科学、纳米技术、生物医学工程、肿瘤学等多个学科领域的知识与技术,展示了跨学科研究在攻克复杂疾病中的巨大潜力与无限魅力。它不仅是一部聚焦近红外多功能纳米探针在胃肠道恶性肿瘤诊疗应用的专业著作,更是一本引领读者领略多学科协同创新风采、拓宽学术视野的佳作。相信本书的问世,将有力促进近红外多功能纳米探针技术在胃肠道恶性肿瘤领域的深入研究与广泛应用,为提升我国乃至全球在该领域的诊疗水平作出积极贡献。

杨正阳

目录

第1章 绪论 ········· 001
- 1.1 纳米粒子应用概述 ········· 002
- 1.2 纳米粒子在胃肠道恶性肿瘤诊断中的应用 ········· 003
  - 1.2.1 胃肠道恶性肿瘤的常规诊断及其局限性 ········· 003
  - 1.2.2 纳米粒子在胃肠道恶性肿瘤传统影像学诊断中的应用 ········· 003
  - 1.2.3 纳米粒子在胃肠道恶性肿瘤新型成像中的应用 ········· 006
  - 1.2.4 纳米粒子在胃肠道恶性肿瘤血液学检查中的应用 ········· 008
- 1.3 纳米粒子在胃肠道恶性肿瘤治疗中的应用 ········· 010
  - 1.3.1 胃肠道恶性肿瘤治疗现状及其局限性 ········· 010
  - 1.3.2 纳米粒子载药系统在胃肠道恶性肿瘤治疗中的应用 ········· 011
  - 1.3.3 纳米粒子在抑制胃肠道恶性肿瘤乏氧微环境中的应用 ········· 012
  - 1.3.4 纳米粒子在胃肠道恶性肿瘤其他治疗中的应用 ········· 012
- 1.4 意义及研究内容 ········· 013
  - 1.4.1 意义 ········· 013
  - 1.4.2 研究内容 ········· 013
- 参考文献 ········· 015

第2章 构建线粒体靶向型产氧纳米颗粒实现胃肠道恶性肿瘤的靶向诊断及

增强的光动力治疗 ·· 027
　2.1　引言 ··· 028
　2.2　材料与方法 ··· 030
　　　2.2.1　实验材料与仪器 ·· 030
　　　2.2.2　实验方法 ··· 031
　2.3　结果与讨论 ··· 035
　　　2.3.1　Mn_3O_4@MSNs@IR780 的合成与表征 ···················· 035
　　　2.3.2　Mn_3O_4@MSNs@IR780 的稳定性 ·························· 037
　　　2.3.3　纳米颗粒体外 H_2O_2 分解及响应性 IR780 释放 ········· 037
　　　2.3.4　Mn_3O_4@MSNs@IR780 纳米颗粒的亚细胞定位 ········ 040
　　　2.3.5　胃肠道恶性肿瘤细胞中乏氧的检测 ························ 041
　　　2.3.6　胃肠道恶性肿瘤细胞中 ROS 产量的检测 ················ 041
　　　2.3.7　Mn_3O_4@MSNs@IR780 的体外抗肿瘤治疗效果 ········ 043
　　　2.3.8　活体近红外荧光成像与体内生物分布 ···················· 043
　　　2.3.9　体内胃肠道恶性肿瘤组织乏氧情况的监测 ·············· 046
　　　2.3.10　体内抗肿瘤治疗效果 ·· 047
　　　2.3.11　生物安全分析 ··· 047
　2.4　总结 ··· 048
　参考文献 ·· 050

第 3 章　近红外引导下纳米介导的线粒体呼吸抑制/损伤途径增强胃肠道恶性肿瘤的光疗效果 ·· 055

　3.1　引言 ··· 056
　3.2　材料与方法 ··· 058
　　　3.2.1　实验材料与仪器 ·· 058
　　　3.2.2　实验方法 ··· 059
　3.3　结果与讨论 ··· 064
　　　3.3.1　P-P-I-M 纳米颗粒的合成与表征 ···························· 064
　　　3.3.2　P-P-I-M 纳米颗粒的光疗能力测定 ························ 066

3.3.3　线粒体功能抑制及细胞毒性 ················· 067
　　3.3.4　胃肠道恶性肿瘤细胞中的乏氧情况检测 ········· 067
　　3.3.5　P-P-I-M 纳米颗粒的亚细胞定位 ··············· 070
　　3.3.6　胃肠道恶性肿瘤细胞中 ROS 产量的检测 ········ 071
　　3.3.7　体外抗肿瘤治疗效果 ······················· 072
　　3.3.8　活体近红外荧光成像 ······················· 073
　　3.3.9　光声成像结果 ····························· 074
　　3.3.10　肿瘤部位 PET-CT 结果 ····················· 074
　　3.3.11　肿瘤部位光声成像结果 ····················· 075
　　3.3.12　肿瘤组织 HIF-1α 免疫组化染色结果 ··········· 076
　　3.3.13　体内抗肿瘤治疗效果 ······················ 077
　　3.3.14　生物安全性分析 ·························· 079
3.4　总结 ······································· 080
参考文献 ··· 081

第4章　主动靶向性氧化钨纳米颗粒介导的胃肠道恶性肿瘤双模诊断及热休克抑制的光热治疗 ··· 089

4.1　引言 ······································· 090
4.2　材料与方法 ································· 093
　　4.2.1　实验材料与仪器 ··························· 093
　　4.2.2　实验方法 ································· 094
4.3　结果与讨论 ································· 098
　　4.3.1　iRGD-$W_{18}O_{49}$-17AAG 的合成与表征 ············· 098
　　4.3.2　胃肠道恶性肿瘤细胞的选择性摄取 ··········· 103
　　4.3.3　体内生物分布及活体近红外荧光成像 ········· 103
　　4.3.4　体外 CT 成像结果 ························· 106
　　4.3.5　小鼠体内 CT 成像结果 ····················· 106
　　4.3.6　体外红外热成像结果 ······················· 107
　　4.3.7　小鼠体内红外热成像结果 ··················· 108

    4.3.8 体外抗肿瘤治疗效果 ……………………………… 108

    4.3.9 体内抗肿瘤治疗效果 ……………………………… 110

    4.3.10 生物安全分析 …………………………………… 111

  4.4 结果与讨论 ……………………………………………… 112

  参考文献 ……………………………………………………… 113

附录 主要缩略词表 ………………………………………… 120

后记 ………………………………………………………………… 123

第1章

绪论

1.1 纳米粒子应用概述

在全球范围,胃肠道恶性肿瘤是第三大癌症相关死亡因素[1],如图1-1所示,胃癌男性发病率远高于女性[2]。据中国国家癌症中心2015年统计结果显示:中国预计每年新发679 100例,死亡498 000例[3]。由于早期患者症状不明显,因此大多数病人是在晚期确诊,伴有较高的侵袭性和淋巴结转移风险,生存率不足20%[4]。同时,早期确诊的病人大多数可通过内镜或手术切除,然后进行放疗或化疗,从而使5年生存率达到90%[5]。因此,寻找更为精准的早期诊断方式就显得尤为重要。尽管只能在有限的情况下使用,纳米颗粒在胃肠道恶性肿瘤的诊断中依然具有很大的潜力[6],不仅可增强传统诊断方式的精确性,还可应用于术中诊断以及血液学快速诊断,其中一些甚至已经进入了临床试验阶段[7]。

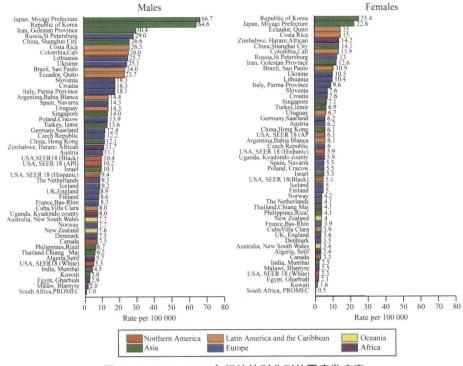

图 1-1 2003—2007 年间按性别分列的胃癌发病率

图片来自参考文献[2]

近年来,随着科学技术的发展,纳米生物这一领域越来越受到人们的关注。纳米生物由于其独特的材料特性,可以增加药物诊断治疗的疗效,降低抗肿瘤药物的毒副作用[8]。目前,许多载药的纳米粒子已被用于胃肠道恶性肿瘤的治疗,例如脂质体阿霉素(Doxil)[9]、聚乙二醇化脂质体阿霉素[10-11]、脂质体紫杉醇[12-13]、白蛋白结合紫杉醇(Abraxane)等[14]。由于不同的理化性质,这些纳米药物具有不同的分布特性和半衰期等,具有很大的应用前景。本节将重点介绍纳米技术在胃肠道恶性肿瘤诊断和治疗中的应用,并讨论其应用前景。

1.2 纳米粒子在胃肠道恶性肿瘤诊断中的应用

1.2.1 胃肠道恶性肿瘤的常规诊断及其局限性

在目前的临床,胃肠道恶性肿瘤的主要诊断方式有三类,即内镜检查、术前影像学检查以及血清学标志物检查,但是,这三种诊断方式均存在各自的一些问题。内镜检查是最重要、最有效的诊断方法,尤其在早期胃肠道恶性肿瘤的诊断中,是临床检查的首选方法[15-16]。但是,内镜检查不足以判断肿瘤侵袭程度以及是否存在淋巴结转移等情况,存在追加手术的可能,会给病人带来二次痛苦和伤害。术前影像学检查主要包括计算机断层扫描(Computed Tomography,CT)、磁共振成像(Magnetic Resonance Imaging,MRI)、正电子发射计算机断层扫描(Positron Emission Computed Tomography,PET-CT)等。然而,影像学诊断主要依据肿瘤组织形态学及代谢的变化,而早期胃肠道恶性肿瘤的形态学及代谢变化均不显著,导致了灵敏度差,难以诊断早期胃肠道恶性肿瘤等一系列问题[17]。血清学标志物主要指肿瘤发生发展过程中产生的化学物质,通常以酶、抗原、蛋白等形式存在,其在肿瘤组织中的含量大大超出正常组织,可用来识别和诊断肿瘤[18]。然而,血清标志物大多经肝脏及胆道排泄,可能导致血清中相关肿瘤标志物浓度过低,降低诊断的灵敏度[19]。同时,一些炎症相关因素也会导致血清标志物浓度升高,进而存在假阳性率过高的问题[20]。因此,解决上述问题,提高胃肠道恶性肿瘤诊断的特异性、灵敏度,并且早期诊断,就显得尤为重要。

1.2.2 纳米粒子在胃肠道恶性肿瘤传统影像学诊断中的应用

近年来,纳米医学的发展为胃肠道恶性肿瘤的影像学诊断开辟了新的途径。由于纳米颗粒特有的尺寸、高载药性、表面可修饰性、可控制释放性以及实体瘤组织的高通透性和滞留(Enhanced Permeability and Retention,EPR)效应(图1-2),可从纳米层面对胃肠道恶性肿瘤进行诊断,解决传统诊断方法的局限性。尽管成功开发一种安全有效并且可用于体内靶向胃肠道恶性肿瘤成像的纳米颗粒是一个巨大的挑战,但一些研究已经在这方面取得了进展。

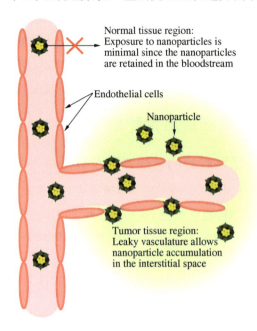

正常组织血管由紧密的内皮细胞排列组成,可防止纳米药物逃逸或外渗。然而肿瘤组织的血管是渗漏的和高渗透的,允许在肿瘤的间质空间优先积聚纳米颗粒,也称为纳米颗粒被动肿瘤靶向。

图 1-2 纳米颗粒在肿瘤组织 EPR 效应示意图

图片来自参考文献[21]

金纳米粒子(Gold Nanoparticles,GNPs)作为一种潜在的 CT 造影剂,近年来得到了广泛的研究。金(Au)化学性质稳定,X 射线质量衰减系数高,同时,GNPs 易于合成,也容易实现表面功能化,进而达到更好的体内效果[22]。Zhang 等人报道了叶酸(Folic acid,FA)共轭谷胱甘肽(Glutathione,GSH)修饰的金纳米簇在胃肠道恶性肿瘤成像中的应用[23]。叶酸在人血清中含量很低,是细胞增殖所必需的维生素,在许多肿瘤细胞表面过表达[24]。这种纳米探针具有良好的生物相容性及稳定性,能够在体外靶向 MGC-803 胃肠道恶性肿瘤细胞系,并且在体内靶向裸鼠荷瘤模型,具有高选择性靶向性。可实现近红外荧光与 CT 多模成像,达到精确诊断的效果。Kukreja 等人报道了基质金属蛋白酶(Matrix Metalloproteinase,MMP)肽包裹金核/氧化铁多孔壳纳米颗粒在胃肠道恶性肿瘤诊断中的应用[25]。基质金属蛋白酶是一种钙-锌离子依赖的蛋白水解酶,在介导肿瘤血管新生、转移和侵袭等过程中发挥重要作用[26]。这种纳米探针由于包裹了 MMP 肽,具有了只在肿瘤组织释放的特性,使得肿瘤部位出现高强度信号。此外,由于金核/氧化铁多孔壳同时具有 T2 对比效应和 X 射线衰减特性,可达到 CT 与 MRI 多模成像的效果,增加了诊断的穿透性与精确度。Shi 等人报道了一种荧光硫化铜(CuS)纳米粒子(RGD-CuS-Cy5.5),能对淋巴结转移性胃肠道恶性肿瘤细胞进行无创近红外荧光与 CT 成像[27],如图 1-3 所示。这种纳米粒子可以通过 $α_vβ_3$ 整合素介导的内吞作用选择性地进入 MKN-45 细胞,同时在体内可以靶向性地进入有转移的前哨淋巴结,有可能实现胃肠道恶性肿瘤的早期诊断以及术中转移性淋巴结的精确清扫。

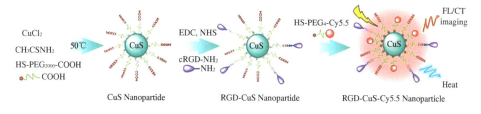

(a) RGD-CuS-Cy5.5 纳米粒的设计合成示意图

该纳米颗粒由强近红外吸收的 CuS 颗粒、敏感的近红外荧光团 Cy5.5 和肿瘤靶向配体 cRGD 组成。

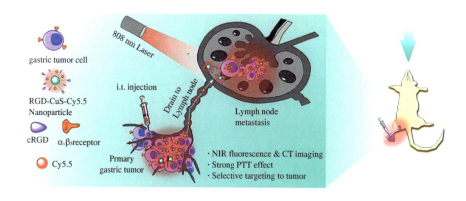

(b) 静脉注射 RGD-CuS-Cy5.5 后,由于纳米颗粒很小,很容易引流到淋巴结

整合素 $α_vβ_3$ 在胃肠道恶性肿瘤细胞中的高表达可通过受体介导的内吞作用触发细胞的有效摄取,并在淋巴结中积聚,从而产生强烈的近红外荧光和 CT 对比度,提示淋巴结转移。

图 1-3 荧光 RGD-CuS-Cy5.5 纳米粒子的设计思路

图片来自参考文献[27]

Yan 等人针对 MRI 报道了利用聚乙二醇(Polyethylene Glycol,PEG)修饰

的四氧化三铁(Fe_3O_4)纳米粒与特异性靶向环肽 GX1 以及近红外荧光染料 Cy5.5 偶联,对胃肠道恶性肿瘤进行磁共振/近红外双模诊断[28]。结果证明,注射纳米粒后的 2~48 h,肿瘤信号强度明显高于背景,同时生物相容性好,具有较好的胃肠道恶性肿瘤靶向聚集效应。Wang 等人用抗 CD146 单克隆抗体[29],Wang 等人用 BRCAA1 单克隆抗体分别标记纳米颗粒用于胃肠道恶性肿瘤的 MRI 成像[30],也取得了不错的效果。曲妥珠单抗是一种人源化单克隆抗体,靶向人表皮生长因子受体 2(Human Epidermal Growth Factor Receptor-2,HER-2)的胞外结构域[31]。曲妥珠单抗是目前唯一被美国食品和药物管理局(Food and Drug Administration,FDA)批准作为 HER-2 阳性转移性胃肠道恶性肿瘤一线治疗的靶点[32]。目前,已有一些曲妥珠单抗共轭的磁性纳米颗粒用于 HER-2 阳性乳腺癌的 MRI 诊断,如超顺磁性氧化铁[33]、荧光超顺磁性氧化铁纳米粒子[34]、铁/中空二氧化硅纳米颗粒(Hs-Fe NPs)等[35]。理论上,这些应用于 HER-2 阳性乳腺癌的纳米粒子也可用于 HER-2 过度表达的胃肠道恶性肿瘤 MRI 诊断[36]。

1.2.3 纳米粒子在胃肠道恶性肿瘤新型成像中的应用

近红外(Near-Infrared,NIR)荧光成像技术是一种在手术过程中实时观察组织形态及代谢的新技术,在术中检测重要解剖结构和肿瘤转移方面具有很强的应用价值。近红外荧光的波长在 700~900 nm 之间,具有很高的组织穿透能力(厘米级别),同时人眼对于近红外波长不敏感,其不会改变手术野的情况[37]。目前,临床上最常使用的近红外光敏剂是美国 FDA 于 1954 年批准的吲哚菁绿(Indocyanine Green,ICG),如图 1-4 所示[38]。静脉注射后,ICG 可在很大程度上(约 98%)与血浆蛋白结合,从而使其不脱离正常血管结构[39]。之后血浆蛋白结合 ICG 主要经由肝脏代谢,因此其可用于胃肠道恶性肿瘤的图像引导下手术[40]。然而,由于光稳定性差、半衰期短和浓度依赖性聚集等问题,ICG 在胃肠道恶性肿瘤的近红外成像受到了很大的限制[41-42]。

针对这一问题,一些 ICG 相关的纳米粒子被设计出来。Tummers 等人使用 ICG 吸附在纳米胶体的方法[43],增加其流体力学直径,如图 1-5 所示,可以使得示踪剂在前哨淋巴结中更好地保留,从而减少二级淋巴结的染色。这一原理已经在乳腺癌和皮肤黑色素瘤中得到了成功的描述[44-45]。在 22 例患者中,有

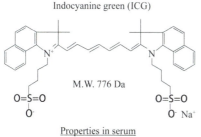
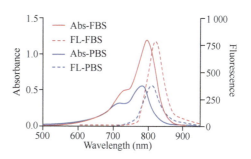

(a) 化学结构和关键光学特性（血清中）

(b) 溶于磷酸盐缓冲液（Phosphate Buffered Saline,PBS）和胎牛血清（Fetal Bovine Serum,FBS）中的 10 μM ICG 的吸收波长和发射波长

图 1-4　ICG 的化学和光学特性

图片来自参考文献[38]

21 例患者至少有 1 个转移淋巴结被近红外荧光成像检测,总准确率为 90%,且准确率随着 pT 分期的升高而降低,对胃肠道恶性肿瘤的手术切除具有重要意义。Hoshino 等人报道了 ICG 脂质体衍生物（LP-ICG-C18）应用于腹膜转移的胃肠道恶性肿瘤猪模型[46]。结果显示,这种近红外荧光脂质体探针能有效地靶向腹膜播散性肿瘤,且易于被近红外成像系统检测,可为胃肠道恶性肿瘤患者提供更精确的诊断方法。此外,载 ICG 乳小体[47]、聚乙二醇脂质体 ICG[48]、整合素介导的 RGD 修饰的聚乙二醇脂质体 ICG 等纳米粒子也被报道用于胃肠道恶性肿瘤的近红外诊断[49-50]。

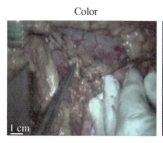
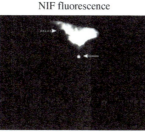
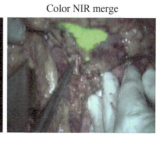

(a) 前哨淋巴结的鉴定

注射 ICG 纳米胶体 ICG:Nanocoll 15 min 后,使用 NIR 荧光成像。肿瘤周围注射部位用虚线箭头表示,前哨淋巴结用实线箭头表示。

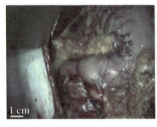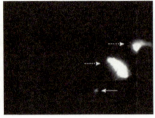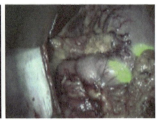

(b) 肿瘤阳性淋巴结患者

注射部位和具有荧光的前哨淋巴结清晰可见。注射部位和淋巴结之间也可见淋巴管。

图 1-5 前哨淋巴结的近红外荧光成像鉴别

图片来自参考文献[43]

另一方面，性能更优于 ICG 的示踪剂也越来越多地被应用于胃肠道恶性肿瘤。IR780 是目前最常用的一种光敏剂，作为一种脂溶性染料，在循环中表现得更稳定，荧光强度更高，保留时间更长，穿透深度更深[51]。Deng 等人报道的使用叶酸连接大分子共轭物包裹 IR780（F-S-C/IR780）[52]，大大提高了 IR780 的溶解性和光稳定性。叶酸受体阳性的胃肠道恶性肿瘤细胞（BGC-823）可有效地吸收 F-S-C/IR780 纳米胶束，进而达到肿瘤主动靶向作用，可用于胃肠道恶性肿瘤的近红外诊断。白蛋白-叶酸复合物包裹 IR780 介孔碳-金杂化纳米探针[53]、氧化锰包裹的 IR780 多孔硅也被报道应用于胃肠道恶性肿瘤的近红外诊断中[54]。

1.2.4 纳米粒子在胃肠道恶性肿瘤血液学检查中的应用

基因组学、蛋白质组学和分子病理学的进展已经产生了许多潜在的胃肠道恶性肿瘤相关血清学生物标志物，其检测也是早期诊断的重要组成部分[55-56]。使用纳米粒子可提高生物标志物的灵敏度，取得更好的效果[57]。纳米颗粒可应用于光学纳米传感器[58]、荧光纳米传感器[59]、电化学纳米传感器[60]、磁性纳米传感器等[61]，可用于检测血清中高表达的糖类抗原 125（Carbohydrate Antigen 125，CA125）[62]、癌胚抗原（Carcinoembryonic Antigen，CEA）[63]、HER-2[64]（图 1-6）等高表达于胃肠道恶性肿瘤患者的血清标志物，因此它们也可用于早期胃肠道恶性肿瘤的初筛检测与诊断。

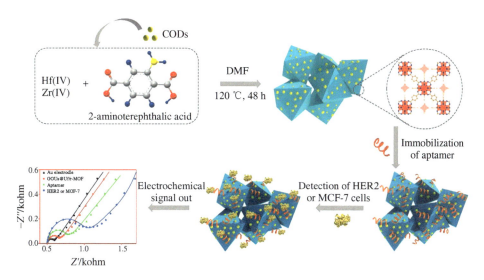

图1-6 用于检测HER2的CDs@ZrHf-MOF传感器的制备过程示意图

图片来自参考文献[64]

循环肿瘤细胞(Circulating Tumor Cells,CTCs)可定义为液体活检,是一种新兴的肿瘤诊断、监测的微创工具。循环肿瘤细胞可用于确定预后,实时监测治疗反应和肿瘤复发,探索治疗目标,以及研究其中的转移癌生物学和耐药机制潜在地开发新药[65-66]。血液中循环肿瘤细胞作为转移性胃肠道恶性肿瘤的诊断、预后和分子检测的潜在生物标志物已被广泛研究[67-68]。由于CTCs在血液中的含量很稀少($10^6 \sim 10^9$ 个血细胞中有1个),因此从血液中高效地捕获循环肿瘤细胞就显得尤为重要[69]。新型的纳米材料由于其自身的特征,在增强循环肿瘤细胞的检测方面具有广阔的应用前景。目前,用于检测或分离CTCs的纳米粒子通常由与循环肿瘤细胞已知生物标记物特异结合的配体和通过特定信号检测或从血液中捕获的纳米粒子两部分组成[70]。利用纳米粒子检测和分离循环肿瘤细胞的研究主要集中在肺癌[71]、乳腺癌[72]、前列腺癌[73]等,而针对胃肠道恶性肿瘤CTCs的报道相对较少。He等人利用TiO_2纳米颗粒组成的生物相容性纳米膜从胃肠道恶性肿瘤患者外周血样本中分离出循环肿瘤细胞,如图1-7所示[74],且由于纳米薄膜具有良好的生物相容性,可对捕获的癌细胞进行原位培养,为捕获细胞数量不足以分析时提供了另一种选择。结果显示,约50%的细胞可以从基质上分离出来,存在潜在临床应用的可能。此外,一些用于检测特殊标记物的纳米颗粒,如CD45[75]、CEA[76]、HER-2等[77],也有望成为胃肠道恶性肿瘤循环肿瘤细胞的潜在检测靶点。

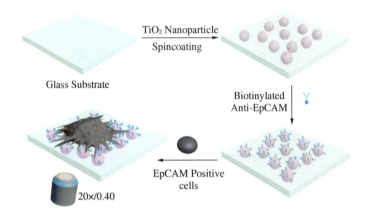

该纳米颗粒通过多步修饰,进而被抗上皮细胞黏着分子抗体包裹,检测阳性的循环肿瘤细胞。

图 1-7 通过介孔 TiO2 纳米颗粒生物检测罕见的循环肿瘤细胞示意图

图片来自参考文献[74]

1.3 纳米粒子在胃肠道恶性肿瘤治疗中的应用

1.3.1 胃肠道恶性肿瘤治疗现状及其局限性

外科手术仍然是胃肠道恶性肿瘤治疗的主要手段,也是唯一可能的根治手段。根治性的胃肠道恶性肿瘤手术不但要完整地对原发病灶进行切除,而且需要彻底地清扫区域淋巴结,包括标准手术、改良手术和扩大手术[78]。然而,早期胃肠道恶性肿瘤多无特殊症状,难以发现,确诊时多已属晚期,手术切除率低,且术后易复发转移,术后 3 年生存率也仅约 10%[79]。除外科手术外,化疗、放疗或免疫治疗的单独治疗以及联合辅助治疗在胃肠道恶性肿瘤中被证明是有益的[80]。对于进展期胃肠道恶性肿瘤,新辅助治疗联合手术比单独手术更为优越,5 年无进展率为 23%～36%[81]。然而,化疗只能用于功能状态评分(Performance Status,PS)表现良好的患者,即 PS≤1[82]。细胞减灭术+腹腔热灌注化疗(HIPEC)也可提高胃源性局限性腹膜癌患者的生存率,但也仅仅局限于腹膜癌指数(Peritoneal Cancer Index,PCI)小于 12 的患者[83-84]。计量控制不当的放疗也有可能在原本正常的组织当中诱发细胞癌变,与治疗的初衷是背道而驰的[85]。因此,依托肿瘤纳米技术,开发更安全、更有效的抗肿瘤治疗手段,改变癌症治疗的现状,就显得尤为重要。

1.3.2 纳米粒子载药系统在胃肠道恶性肿瘤治疗中的应用

纳米载体脂质体是一种双层磷脂囊泡,可将疏水性和亲水性药物包埋在脂质双层中或内部水核中来减少脂质双层的数量,进而将脂质体的尺寸减小到纳米级别,从而增加包裹药物的循环时间和肿瘤定位特性[86]。Cascinu 等人的随机Ⅱ期临床试验证明,脂质体阿霉素、顺铂和 5-氟尿嘧啶联合用药有效率明显高于任何阿霉素,同时具有很好的安全性[10]。Recchia 等人评估了使用聚乙二醇脂质体阿霉素与奥沙利铂联用对于早期接受化疗的转移性胃肠道恶性肿瘤患者的疗效和安全性[11]。结果证明,这种化疗方案是一种有效的治疗方案,同时可以缓解大部分转移性胃肠道恶性肿瘤患者接受多西紫杉醇后的毒副反应症状。

可生物降解的聚合物如聚乳酸、白蛋白、壳聚糖等,因其可控缓释性能、亚细胞大小和生物相容性而得到了广泛的应用,如图 1-8 所示[87]。白蛋白结合紫杉醇(Abraxane)目前已被 FDA 批准用于治疗不能手术患者或放疗患者的局部晚期转移性肿瘤[88]。Van De Sande 等人通过临床前和早期临床试验结果证明,白蛋白结合紫杉醇比标准溶剂紫杉醇在治疗腹膜转移肿瘤方面具有更好的疗效,可应用于胃肠道恶性肿瘤腹膜转移患者的治疗[14]。

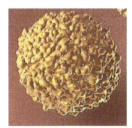
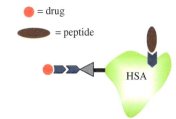

(a) 药物与人白蛋白血清物理结合并形成药物纳米粒子　　(b) 白蛋白结合肽或前药经静脉注射并原位结合到循环白蛋白上

图 1-8　白蛋白作为药物载体示意图

图片来自参考文献[87]

介孔二氧化硅纳米粒(Mesoporous Silica Nanoparticles,MSNs)由于其载药的动态能力、药物的可控制释放性以及多功能性,在抗癌药物的缓释研究中得到了越来越广泛的应用[89]。Naz 等人使用介孔二氧化硅包裹阿霉素,发现其具有良好的抗肿瘤活性,但对正常细胞的毒性要低得多,有很强的靶向肿瘤治疗潜力[90]。

1.3.3 纳米粒子在抑制胃肠道恶性肿瘤乏氧微环境中的应用

近年来,越来越多的证据表明,肿瘤不仅是一个宏观的肿块,而且是一个复杂的组织,涉及极其复杂的微环境成分。低氧环境下的肿瘤乏氧微环境已被广泛证实,可通过抑制药物疗效,限制肿瘤免疫细胞浸润,进而加速肿瘤的复发和转移,降低肿瘤治疗的疗效[91]。Cheng 等人使用全氟化碳囊泡(图 1-9)[92],Zhou 等人使用血红蛋白用作纳米载体以直接将氧输送到低氧环境中[93],均取得了一定的效果。Liu 等人使用金纳米团簇[94],Song 等人使用二氧化锰纳米粒子分解肿瘤内部过表达的过氧化氢(H_2O_2)生成氧气[95],解决肿瘤局部的乏氧微环境。尽管这方面研究涉及胃肠道恶性肿瘤较少,但理论上,上述纳米颗粒同样适用于胃肠道恶性肿瘤乏氧微环境的改善及治疗。

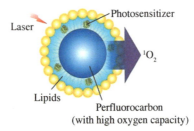

光敏剂和全氟化碳是由脂类共同包裹的。光敏剂均匀地分散在脂质单分子层中,而全氟化碳则分散在纳米粒子的核心。同时,在激光照射下,光敏剂可将能量转移到富含氧气的全氟化碳中,产生活性氧自由基,从而增强肿瘤抑制作用。

图 1-9 全氟化碳囊泡纳米颗粒结构示意图

图片来自参考文献[92]

1.3.4 纳米粒子在胃肠道恶性肿瘤其他治疗中的应用

自噬,能促进循环中不活跃的肿瘤细胞和增殖癌细胞的存在,促进肿瘤细胞干细胞样亚群的存在,进而诱导肿瘤细胞的侵袭和放射抗性[96-97]。近年来的研究证明,纳米颗粒具有自噬控制特性,可在不同的自噬相关肿瘤的治疗中提供良好的应用潜力[98]。Li 等人报道了海藻酸钠包裹的 Fe_3O_4 磁性纳米粒子可通过诱导细胞自噬和凋亡,显著抑制多药耐药胃肿瘤的生长,降低肿瘤体积,机制可能与线粒体功能紊乱和 ROS 过度积累有关[99]。

基因治疗是通过将 DNA、RNA、siRNA 等遗传物质转移到细胞中,纠正正常蛋白质的产生,可以达到肿瘤治疗的目的。其重点是刺激对肿瘤的保护性免疫反应、替换突变的肿瘤抑制基因及骨髓/外周血干细胞中的多药耐药基因等[100]。由于纳米颗粒可以提供增强的细胞摄取、更深的组织渗透性和特定细胞类型的靶向性,且核酸结构在细胞和血液中的降解时间较短,因此选择纳米颗粒作为给药途径在基因传递中非常重要[101]。Huo 通过壳聚糖包裹 BRAF 的 siRNA 纳米粒,下调胃肠道恶性肿瘤细胞 BRAF 的表达,明显降低了胃肠道恶性肿瘤的侵袭能力[102]。

1.4 意义及研究内容

1.4.1 意义

在过去的十年中,胃肠道恶性肿瘤是全球最常见的恶性肿瘤。然而,由于胃肠道恶性肿瘤早期的无症状性,诊断上的延迟会导致胃肠道恶性肿瘤进展到晚期时才被确诊,因为侵犯邻近组织和转移等原因,限制了手术的有效性。同时,针对晚期胃肠道恶性肿瘤病人,化疗的客观有效率只有不到 40%,化疗后中位总生存期只有不到 11 个月,此外,化疗的严重副作用也不容忽视。

自问世以来,纳米技术在生物技术和医疗领域的应用越来越受到关注。纳米医学可以为胃肠道恶性肿瘤的诊断与治疗提供许多潜在包括成像和治疗在内的许多好处,包括胃肠道恶性肿瘤的早期检测、被动和主动病灶靶向、增强药物的生物相容性,同时进行疾病治疗和监测。纳米材料在胃肠道恶性肿瘤的应用中主要包括以下优势:① 纳米颗粒可以被生物分子功能化,使其能够靶向肿瘤组织,定位于目标病灶;② 纳米颗粒通常可以通过表面修饰,包裹或添加配方来克服普通化疗药物溶解性和稳定性的问题;③ 纳米颗粒具有新颖的物理性质,如近红外荧光成像、光声成像等,可用于生物成像;④ 纳米颗粒通常由数千个具有高表面积的物质组成,因此可以携带更高的治疗载荷,对于肿瘤组织的杀伤更为严重;⑤ 纳米颗粒可通过被动或主动靶向,在肿瘤部位有效累积,从而显著降低器官非特异性毒性。

本节针对目前胃肠道恶性肿瘤早期诊断所遇到的问题,结合晚期治疗副作用严重及预后差的问题,应用纳米医学技术,设计制备可用于胃肠道恶性肿瘤诊断与治疗一体化的多功能纳米颗粒,通过对胃肠道恶性肿瘤的靶向成像,联合光疗,为解决目前胃肠道恶性肿瘤的诊断与治疗困境提供了新的思路。

1.4.2 研究内容

研究内容主要分为以下三个部分:

(1) 设计制备一种多功能纳米复合材料(Mn_3O_4@MSNs@IR780),可以同时实现近红外下的胃肠道恶性肿瘤诊断以及氧气释放下线粒体靶向的胃肠道恶性肿瘤增强光动力治疗。四氧化三锰(Mn_3O_4)作为门卫,阻断载有光敏剂(IR780)的多孔硅(MSNs)通道。Mn_3O_4@MSNs@IR780 纳米颗粒可通过EPR效应有效地靶向胃肠道恶性肿瘤组织,其中 Mn_3O_4 作为一种有效的催化剂,可以持续地将胃肠道恶性肿瘤局部高表达的 H_2O_2 分解,产生氧气,同时崩解导致 MSNs 通道的打开;IR780 在肿瘤组织中释放,进一步靶向线粒体,在 808 nm 波长的激光照射下,在线粒体附近生成活性氧(Reactive Oxygen Species,ROS),损伤线粒体,进而杀伤胃肠道恶性肿瘤组织。同时,IR780 作为一种光敏剂,可以准确地检测肿瘤的位置。

(2) 使用两亲性的聚乙二醇(PEG)聚己内酯(Polycaprolactone,PCL)包裹光敏剂(IR780)以及二甲双胍(Metformin,MET),合成一种可以同时实现近红外下的胃肠道恶性肿瘤诊断,以及内源性乏氧抑制和线粒体靶向胃肠道恶性肿瘤光动力疗法(Photodynamic Therapy,PDT)/光热疗法(Photothermal Therapy,PTT)的多功能纳米颗粒 PEG-PCL-IR780-MET(P-P-I-M)。PEG-PCL 作为纳米载体,具有较高的稳定性,并通过 EPR 效应将纳米颗粒靶向传递到胃肠道恶性肿瘤组织中。一旦纳米颗粒在肿瘤组织中积聚,808 nm 波长的激光可进一步释放二甲双胍和 IR780。二甲双胍可直接抑制线粒体电子传递链中的还原型烟酰胺腺嘌呤二核苷酸(Nicotinamide Adenine Dinucleotide,NADH)脱氢酶的活性,从而实现对细胞呼吸的有效抑制,改善肿瘤乏氧微环境;光敏剂 IR780 迅速靶向线粒体,产生活性氧并产热,发挥线粒体靶向 PDT 和 PTT 的协同治疗效果。另外,基于 IR780 的光声(Photoacoustic,PA)和 NIR 双模态成像特性,研究人员可以通过近红外/光声双模成像监测 PDT 及 PTT 的协同作用,发现微小肿瘤灶。

(3) 设计制备了一种包含羧基功能化氧化钨($W_{18}O_{49}$)、整合素靶向多肽(iRGD)和热休克蛋白 90(Heat Shock Protein,HSP90)抑制剂坦螺旋霉素(Tanespimycin,17AAG)的纳米颗粒(iRGD-$W_{18}O_{49}$-17AAG),可有效增强纳米颗粒对于胃肠道恶性肿瘤组织的靶向性以及成像的穿透性,提高其在胃肠道恶性肿瘤诊断与治疗中的应用。$W_{18}O_{49}$ 含有活性羧基基团且具有较高的光热性能和较高的体内外生物安全性,可作为光热治疗的载体。同时,由于含有钨这种金属元素,其具有强大的 X 射线吸收能力,可作为 CT 的造影剂。新型 N 端半胱氨酸环型多肽 iRGD 相较于传统的精氨酸-甘氨酸-天冬氨酸（Arginine-Glycine-Aspartic，RGD）多肽，保留了整合素靶向性，同时提升了肿瘤细胞的穿透性。17AAG 可以通过酯化作用与 $W_{18}O_{49}$ 结合，抑制胃肠道恶性肿瘤细胞的热休克反应，提高了光热治疗的疗效。同时，使用染料 Cy5.5 修饰 iRGD-$W_{18}O_{49}$-17AAG 纳米颗粒，可以通过 CT/NIR 近红外荧光双模成像寻找胃肠道恶性肿瘤病灶并监测纳米颗粒的体内外生物分布。

参考文献

[1] ALLEMANI C, WEIR H K, CARREIRA H, et al. Global surveillance of cancer survival 1995—2009：analysis of individual data for 25,676,887 patients from 279 population-based registries in 67 countries(CONCORD-2). Lancet, 2015, 385(9972):977-1010.

[2] TORRE L A, SIEGEL R L, WARD E M, et al. Global cancer incidence and mortality rates and trends：an update. Cancer Epidemiol Biomarkers Prev, 2016, 25(1):16-27.

[3] CHEN W, ZHENG R, BAADE P D, et al. Cancer statistics in China, 2015. CA Cancer J Clin., 2016, 66(2):115-132.

[4] ROVIELLO G, CONTER F U, MINI E, et al. Nanoparticle albumin-bound paclitaxel：a big nano for the treatment of gastric cancer. Cancer Chemother Pharmacol, 2019, 84(4):669-677.

[5] YOKOYAMA T, KAMADA K, TSURUI Y, et al. Clinicopathological analysis for recurrence of stage Ib gastric cancer(according to the second English edition of the Japanese classification of gastric carcinoma). Gastric Cancer, 2011, 14(4):372-377.

[6] EOM G, KIM H, HWANG A, et al. Nanogap-Rich Au Nanowire SERS sensor for ultrasensitive telomerase activity detection：Application to gastric and breast cancer tissues diagnosis. Advanced Functional Materials, 2017, 27(37):1701832.

[7] WANG Y X. Superparamagnetic iron oxide based MRI contrast agents：Current status of clinical application. Quant Imaging Med Surg., 2011, 1(1):35-40.

[8] RILEY R S, JUNE C H, LANGER R, et al. Delivery technologies for cancer immunotherapy. Nat Rev Drug Discov., 2019, 18(3):175-196.

[9] BEYER I, CAO H, PERSSON J, et al. Coadministration of epithelial junction opener JO-1 improves the efficacy and safety of chemotherapeutic drugs. Clin Cancer Res., 2012, 18(12):3340-3351.

[10] CASCINU S, GALIZIA E, LABIANCA R, et al. Pegylated liposomal doxorubicin, 5-fluorouracil and cisplatin versus mitomycin-C, 5-fluorouracil and cisplatin for advanced gastric cancer: a randomized phase II trial. Cancer Chemother Pharmacol, 2011, 68(1):37-43.

[11] RECCHIA F, CANDELORO G, GUERRIERO G, et al. Liposomal pegylated doxorubicin and oxaliplatin as salvage chemotherapy in patients with metastatic gastric cancer treated earlier. Anticancer Drugs, 2010, 21(5):559-564.

[12] CHEN L, CHEN Q, ZHUANG Z, et al. Effect of the weekly administration of liposome-Paclitaxel combined with s-1 on advanced gastric cancer. Jpn J Clin Oncol., 2014, 44(3):208-213.

[13] XU X, WANG L, XU H Q, et al. Clinical comparison between paclitaxel liposome (Lipusu®) and paclitaxel for treatment of patients with metastatic gastric cancer. Asian Pac J Cancer Prev., 2013, 14(4):2591-2594.

[14] VAN DE SANDE L, GRAVERSEN M, HUBNER M, et al. Intraperitoneal aerosolization of albumin-stabilized paclitaxel nanoparticles (Abraxane™) for peritoneal carcinomatosis: a phase I first-in-human study. Pleura Peritoneum, 2018, 3(2):20180112.

[15] CHOI I J, KOOK M C, KIM Y I, et al. Helicobacter pylori therapy for the prevention of metachronous gastric cancer. N Engl J Med., 2018, 378(12):1085-1095.

[16] ONO H, YAO K, FUJISHIRO M, et al. Guidelines for endoscopic submucosal dissection and endoscopic mucosal resection for early gastric cancer. Dig Endosc., 2016, 28(1):3-15.

[17] LIU S, GUAN W, WANG H, et al. Apparent diffusion coefficient value of gastric cancer by diffusion-weighted imaging: correlations with the

histological differentiation and Lauren classification. Eur J Radiol., 2014, 83(12):2122-2128.

[18] LIU H, ZHU L, LIU B, et al. Genome-wide microRNA profiles identify miR-378 as a serum biomarker for early detection of gastric cancer. Cancer Lett., 2012, 316(2):196-203.

[19] ZHANG Z, DOU M, YAO X, et al. Potential biomarkers in diagnosis of human gastric cancer. Cancer Invest, 2016, 34(3):115-122.

[20] OHTSUKA T, SATO S, KITAJIMA Y, et al. False-positive findings for tumor markers after curative gastrectomy for gastric cancer. Dig Dis Sci., 2008, 53(1):73-79.

[21] NIE S, XING Y, KIM G J, et al. Nanotechnology applications in cancer. Annu Rev Biomed Eng., 2007: 257-288.

[22] WANG H, LI S, ZHANG L, et al. Tunable fabrication of folic acid-Au@poly(acrylic acid)/mesoporous calcium phosphate Janus nanoparticles for CT imaging and active-targeted chemotherapy of cancer cells. Nanoscale, 2017, 9(38):14322-14326.

[23] ZHANG C, ZHOU Z, QIAN Q, et al. Glutathione-capped fluorescent gold nanoclusters for dual-modal fluorescence/X-ray computed tomography imaging. J Mater Chem B., 2013, 1(38):5045-5053.

[24] PARK J, JIANG Q, FENG D, et al. Size-Controlled Synthesis of Porphyrinic Metal-Organic Framework and Functionalization for Targeted Photodynamic Therapy. J Am Chem Soc., 2016, 138(10):3518-3525.

[25] KUKREJA A, KANG B, KIM H O, et al. Preparation of Gold Core-Mesoporous Iron-Oxide Shell Nanoparticles and their application as dual MR/CT contrast agent in human gastric cancer cells. Journal of Industrial & Engineering Chemistry, 2017, 48:56-65.

[26] MA T, HOU Y, ZENG J, et al. Dual-ratiometric target-triggered fluorescent probe for simultaneous quantitative visualization of tumor microenvironment protease activity and pH in vivo. J Am Chem Soc., 2018, 140(1):211-218.

[27] SHI H, YAN R, WU L, et al. Tumor-targeting CuS nanoparticles for

multimodal imaging and guided photothermal therapy of lymph node metastasis. Acta Biomater. , 2018, 72:256 - 265.

[28] YAN X, SONG X, WANG Z. Construction of specific magnetic resonance imaging/optical dual-modality molecular probe used for imaging angiogenesis of gastric cancer. Artif Cells Nanomed Biotechnol, 2017, 45(3):399 - 403.

[29] WANG P, QU Y, LI C, et al. Bio-functionalized dense-silica nanoparticles for MR/NIRF imaging of CD146 in gastric cancer. Int J Nanomedicine. , 2015, 10:749 - 763.

[30] WANG K, RUAN J, QIAN Q, et al. BRCAA1 monoclonal antibody conjugated fluorescent magnetic nanoparticles for in vivo targeted magnetofluorescent imaging of gastric cancer. J Nanobiotechnology. , 2011, 9:23.

[31] VON MINCKWITZ G, HUANG C S, MANO M S, et al. Trastuzumab emtansine for residual invasive HER2-positive breast cancer. N Engl J Med. , 2019, 380(7):617 - 628.

[32] SHI J, LI F, YAO X, et al. The HER4-YAP1 axis promotes trastuzumab resistance in HER2-positive gastric cancer by inducing epithelial and mesenchymal transition. Oncogene, 2018, 37(22):3022 - 3038.

[33] ALRIC C, AUBREY N, ALLARD-VANNIER E, et al. Covalent conjugation of cysteine-engineered scFv to PEGylated magnetic nanoprobes for immunotargeting of breast cancer cells. Rsc Advances, 2016, 6(43):37099 - 37109.

[34] LI D L, TAN J E, TIAN Y, et al. Multifunctional superparamagnetic nanoparticles conjugated with fluorescein-labeled designed ankyrin repeat protein as an efficient HER2-targeted probe in breast cancer. Biomaterials, 2017, 147:86 - 98.

[35] LI X, XIA S, ZHOU W, et al. Targeted Fe-doped silica nanoparticles as a novel ultrasound-magnetic resonance dual-mode imaging contrast agent for HER2-positive breast cancer. Int J Nanomedicine. , 2019, 14:2397 - 2413.

[36] LI R, LIU B, GAO J. The application of nanoparticles in diagnosis and

theranostics of gastric cancer. Cancer Lett., 2017, 386:123-130.

[37] BONI L, DAVID G, MANGANO A, et al. Clinical applications of indocyanine green(ICG) enhanced fluorescence in laparoscopic surgery. Surg Endosc, 2015, 29(7):2046-2055.

[38] SCHAAFSMA B E, MIEOG J S, HUTTEMAN M, et al. The clinical use of indocyanine green as a near-infrared fluorescent contrast agent for image-guided oncologic surgery. J Surg Oncol., 2011, 104(3):323-332.

[39] LAU C T, AU D M, WONG K K Y. Application of indocyanine green in pediatric surgery. Pediatr Surg Int., 2019, 35(10):1035-1041.

[40] TAKEUCHI H, KITAGAWA Y. Sentinel node navigation surgery in patients with early gastric cancer. Dig Surg., 2013, 30(2):104-111.

[41] WANG H, LI X, TSE B W, et al. Indocyanine green-incorporating nanoparticles for cancer theranostics. Theranostics, 2018, 8(5):1227-1242.

[42] WANG Y W, FU Y Y, PENG Q, et al. Dye-enhanced graphene oxide for photothermal therapy and photoacoustic imaging. J Mater Chem B., 2013, 1(42):5762-5767.

[43] TUMMERS Q R, BOOGERD L S, DE STEUR W O, et al. Near-infrared fluorescence sentinel lymph node detection in gastric cancer: A pilot study. World J Gastroenterol., 2016, 22(13):3644-3651.

[44] SCHAAFSMA B E, VERBEEK F P, RIETBERGEN D D, et al. Clinical trial of combined radio-and fluorescence-guided sentinel lymph node biopsy in breast cancer. Br J Surg., 2013, 100(8):1037-1044.

[45] BROUWER O R, KLOP W M, BUCKLE T, et al. Feasibility of sentinel node biopsy in head and neck melanoma using a hybrid radioactive and fluorescent tracer. Ann Surg Oncol., 2012, 19(6):1988-1994.

[46] HOSHINO I, MARUYAMA T, FUJITO H, et al. Detection of peritoneal dissemination with near-infrared fluorescence laparoscopic imaging using a liposomal formulation of a synthesized indocyanine green liposomal derivative. Anticancer Res., 2015, 35(3):1353-1359.

[47] TSUJIMOTO H, MORIMOTO Y, TAKAHATA R, et al. Photodynamic therapy using nanoparticle loaded with indocyanine green for experimen-

tal peritoneal dissemination of gastric cancer. Cancer Sci., 2014, 105(12):1626 – 1630.

[48] TSUJIMOTO H,MORIMOTO Y,TAKAHATA R,et al. Theranostic photosensitive nanoparticles for lymph node metastasis of gastric cancer. Ann Surg Oncol., 2015, 22(Suppl 3):S923 – S928.

[49] LOZANO N,AL-AHMADY Z S,BEZIERE N S,et al. Monoclonal antibody-targeted PEGylated liposome-ICG encapsulating doxorubicin as a potential theranostic agent. Int J Pharm., 2015, 482(1/2):2 – 10.

[50] DING J,FENG M,WANG F,et al. Targeting effect of PEGylated liposomes modified with the Arg-Gly-Asp sequence on gastric cancer. Oncol Rep., 2015, 34(4):1825 – 1834.

[51] ZHANG L,WANG D,YANG K,et al. Mitochondria-Targeted Artificial "Nano-RBCs" for Amplified Synergistic Cancer Phototherapy by a Single NIR Irradiation. Adv Sci., 2018, 5(8):1800049.

[52] DENG L, GUO W, LI G, et al. Hydrophobic IR780 loaded sericin nanomicelles for phototherapy with enhanced antitumor efficiency. Int J Pharm., 2019, 566:549 – 556.

[53] ZHANG A,PAN S,ZHANG Y,et al. Carbon-gold hybrid nanoprobes for real-time imaging,photothermal/photodynamic and nanozyme oxidative therapy. Theranostics, 2019, 9(12):3443 – 3458.

[54] YANG Z,WANG J,AI S,et al. Self-generating oxygen enhanced mitochondrion-targeted photodynamic therapy for tumor treatment with hypoxia scavenging. Theranostics, 2019, 9(23):6809 – 6823.

[55] SEIDLITZ T,MERKER S R,ROTHE A,et al. Human gastric cancer modelling using organoids. Gut., 2019, 68(2):207 – 217.

[56] HAN D,LI J,WANG H,et al. Circular RNA circMTO1 acts as the sponge of microRNA-9 to suppress hepatocellular carcinoma progression. Hepatology, 2017, 66(4):1151 – 1164.

[57] LUDWIG J A,WEINSTEIN J N. Biomarkers in cancer staging,prognosis and treatment selection. Nat Rev Cancer., 2005, 5(11):845 – 856.

[58] ZHENG X,TANG H,XIE C,et al. Tracking cancer metastasis in vivo by

using an iridium-based hypoxia-activated optical oxygen nanosensor. Angew Chem Int Ed Engl. , 2015, 54(28):8094 – 8099.

[59] LU L, TU D, LIU Y, et al. Ultrasensitive detection of cancer biomarker microRNA by amplification of fluorescence of lanthanide nanoprobes. Nano Research, 2018, 11(1): 264 – 273.

[60] FU Y, WANG N, YANG A, et al. Highly sensitive detection of protein biomarkers with organic electrochemical transistors. Adv Mater. , 2017, 29(41): 201703787.

[61] TAVALLAIE R, MCCARROLL J, LE GRAND M, et al. Nucleic acid hybridization on an electrically reconfigurable network of gold-coated magnetic nanoparticles enables microRNA detection in blood. Nat Nanotechnol. , 2018, 13(11):1066 – 1071.

[62] CHAKKARAPANI S K, ZHANG P, AHN S, et al. Total internal reflection plasmonic scattering-based fluorescence-free nanoimmunosensor probe for ultra-sensitive detection of cancer antigen 125. Biosens Bioelectron, 2016, 81:23 – 31.

[63] LI X, SUN M, CHEN B, et al. A split organic photophotochemical transistor/vision sensing platform based on MNZ composite and ZIF-67/CuCoO nanospheres for ultra-sensitive detection of CEA. Biosens Bioelectron, 2025, 268:116896.

[64] GU C, GUO C, LI Z, et al. Bimetallic ZrHf-based metal-organic framework embedded with carbon dots: ultra-sensitive platform for early diagnosis of HER2 and HER2-overexpressed living cancer cells. Biosens Bioelectron, 2019, 134:8 – 15.

[65] FERREIRA M M, RAMANI V C, JEFFREY S S. Circulating tumor cell technologies. Mol Oncol. , 2016, 10(3):374 – 394.

[66] SMALL A C, GONG Y, OH W K, et al. The emerging role of circulating tumor cell detection in genitourinary cancer. J Urol. , 2012, 188(1): 21 – 26.

[67] Beeharry M K, Liu W T, Yan M, et al. New blood markers detection technology: a leap in the diagnosis of gastric cancer. World J Gastroen-

terol, 2016, 22(3):1202-1212.

[68] DE MATTOS-ARRUDA L, OLMOS D, TABERNERO J. Prognostic and predictive roles for circulating biomarkers in gastrointestinal cancer. Future Oncol, 2011, 7(12):1385-1397.

[69] HONG B, ZU Y. Detecting circulating tumor cells: current challenges and new trends. Theranostics, 2013, 3(6):377-394.

[70] LEE H J, CHO H Y, OH J H, et al. Simultaneous capture and in situ analysis of circulating tumor cells using multiple hybrid nanoparticles. Biosens Bioelectron, 2013, 47:508-514.

[71] WANG C, YE M, CHENG L, et al. Simultaneous isolation and detection of circulating tumor cells with a microfluidic silicon-nanowire-array integrated with magnetic upconversion nanoprobes. Biomaterials, 2015, 54:55-62.

[72] BHATTACHARYYA K, GOLDSCHMIDT B S, HANNINK M, et al. Gold nanoparticle-mediated detection of circulating cancer cells. Clin Lab Med., 2012, 32(1):89-101.

[73] ZHANG Y, ZHANG F, SONG Y, et al. Interfacial Polymerization Produced Magnetic Particles with Nano-Filopodia for Highly Accurate Liquid Biopsy in the PSA Gray Zone. Adv Mater., 2023, 35(48):e2303821.

[74] HE R, ZHAO L, LIU Y, et al. Biocompatible TiO_2 nanoparticle-based cell immunoassay for circulating tumor cells capture and identification from cancer patients. Biomed Microdevices, 2013, 15(4):617-626.

[75] CHENG B, WANG S, CHEN Y, et al. A Combined negative and positive enrichment assay for cancer cells isolation and purification. Technol Cancer Res T., 2016, 15(1):69-76.

[76] Zhang H, Fu X, Hu J, et al. Microfluidic bead-based multienzyme-nanoparticle amplification for detection of circulating tumor cells in the blood using quantum dots labels. Anal Chim Acta., 2013;779:64-71.

[77] HUERTA-NUÑEZ L F E, GUTIERREZ-IGLESIAS G, MARTINEZ-CUAZITL A, et al. A biosensor capable of identifying low quantities of breast cancer cells by electrical impedance spectroscopy. Sci Rep.,

2019, 9(1):6419.

[78] CATS A, JANSEN EPM, VAN GRIEKEN NCT, et al. Chemotherapy versus chemoradiotherapy after surgery and preoperative chemotherapy for resectable gastric cancer (CRITICS): an international, open-label, randomised phase 3 trial. Lancet Oncol., 2018, 19(5):616-628.

[79] Ebinger S M, Warschkow R, Tarantino I, et al. Modest overall survival improvements from 1998 to 2009 in metastatic gastric cancer patients: a population-based SEER analysis. Gastric Cancer, 2016, 19(3):723-734.

[80] Janunger K G, Hafström L, Nygren P, et al. A systematic overview of chemotherapy effects in gastric cancer. Acta Oncol., 2001, 40(2/3):309-326.

[81] CUNNINGHAM D, ALLUM W H, STENNING S P, et al. Perioperative chemotherapy versus surgery alone for resectable gastroesophageal cancer. N Engl J Med., 2006, 355(1):11-20.

[82] JAPANESE GASTRIC CANCER ASSOCIATION. Japanese gastric cancer treatment guidelines 2014 (ver. 4). Gastric Cancer, 2017, 20(1):1-19.

[83] YANG X J, HUANG C Q, SUO T, et al. Cytoreductive surgery and hyperthermic intraperitoneal chemotherapy improves survival of patients with peritoneal carcinomatosis from gastric cancer: final results of a phase III randomized clinical trial. Ann Surg Oncol., 2011, 18(6):1575-1581.

[84] GLEHEN O, GILLY F N, ARVIEUX C, et al. Peritoneal carcinomatosis from gastric cancer: a multi-institutional study of 159 patients treated by cytoreductive surgery combined with perioperative intraperitoneal chemotherapy. Ann Surg Oncol., 2010, 17(9):2370-2377.

[85] DEARNALEY D P, KHOO V S, NORMAN A R, et al. Comparison of radiation side-effects of conformal and conventional radiotherapy in prostate cancer: a randomised trial. Lancet, 1999, 353(9149):267-272.

[86] PRIDGEN E M, LANGER R, FAROKHZAD O C. Biodegradable, polymeric nanoparticle delivery systems for cancer therapy. Nanomedicine (Lond), 2007, 2(5):669-680.

[87] KRATZ F. A clinical update of using albumin as a drug vehicle: a com-

mentary. J Control Release., 2014, 190:331-336.

[88] BAE K H, LEE J Y, LEE S H, et al. Optically traceable solid lipid nanoparticles loaded with siRNA and paclitaxel for synergistic chemotherapy with in situ imaging. Adv Healthc Mater., 2013, 2(4):576-584.

[89] REN S, YANG J, MA L, et al. Ternary-responsive drug delivery with activatable dual mode contrast-enhanced in vivo imaging. ACS Appl Mater Inter., 2018, 10(38):31947-31958.

[90] NAZ S, WANG M, HAN Y, et al. Enzyme-responsive mesoporous silica nanoparticles for tumor cells and mitochondria multistage-targeted drug delivery. Int J Nanomedicine., 2019, 14:2533-2542.

[91] HU D, CHEN L, QU Y, et al. Oxygen-generating hybrid polymeric nanoparticles with encapsulated doxorubicin and chlorin e6 for trimodal imaging-guided combined chemo-photodynamic therapy. Theranostics, 2018, 8(6):1558-1574.

[92] CHENG Y, CHENG H, JIANG C, et al. Perfluorocarbon nanoparticles enhance reactive oxygen levels and tumour growth inhibition in photodynamic therapy. Nat Commun., 2015, 6:8785.

[93] ZHOU Y L, LI Y M, H E W T. Oxygen-laden mesenchymal stem cells enhance the effect of gastric cancer chemotherapy in vitro. Oncol Lett., 2019, 17(1):1245-1252.

[94] LIU C P, WU T H, LIU C Y, et al. Self-supplying O_2 through the catalase-like activity of gold nanoclusters for photodynamic therapy against hypoxic cancer cells. Small., 2017, 13(26):201700278.

[95] SONG M, LIU T, SHI C, et al. Bioconjugated manganese dioxide nanoparticles enhance chemotherapy response by priming tumor-associated macrophages toward M1-like phenotype and attenuating tumor hypoxia. ACS Nano., 2016, 10(1):633-647.

[96] SOSA M S, BRAGADO P, AGUIRRE-GHISO J A. Mechanisms of disseminated cancer cell dormancy: an awakening field. Nat Rev Cancer., 2014, 14(9):611-622.

[97] PENG Y F, SHI Y H, DING Z B, et al. Autophagy inhibition suppresses

pulmonary metastasis of HCC in mice via impairing anoikis resistance and colonization of HCC cells. Autophagy, 2013, 9(12):2056-2068.

[98] RAJU G S R, PAVITRA E, MERCHANT N, et al. Targeting autophagy in gastrointestinal malignancy by using nanomaterials as drug delivery systems. Cancer Lett., 2018, 419:222-232.

[99] LI X, FENG J, ZHANG R, et al. Quaternized chitosan/alginate-Fe_3O_4 magnetic nanoparticles enhance the chemosensitization of multidrug-resistant gastric carcinoma by regulating cell autophagy activity in mice. J Biomed Nanotechnol., 2016, 12(5):948-961.

[100] HALLAJ-NEZHADI S, DASS C R, LOTFIPOUR F. Intraperitoneal delivery of nanoparticles for cancer gene therapy. Future Oncol., 2013, 9(1):59-68.

[101] HALLAJ-NEZHADI S, VALIZADEH H, DASTMALCHI S, et al. Preparation of chitosan-plasmid DNA nanoparticles encoding interleukin-12 and their expression in CT-26 colon carcinoma cells. J Pharm Pharm Sci., 2011, 14(2):181-195.

[102] HUO J. Effects of chitosan nanoparticle-mediated BRAF siRNA interference on invasion and metastasis of gastric cancer cells. Artif Cells Nanomed Biotechnol, 2016, 44(5):1232-1235.

第 2 章

构建线粒体靶向型产氧纳米颗粒实现胃肠道恶性肿瘤的靶向诊断及增强的光动力治疗

2.1 引言

胃肠道恶性肿瘤是世界上最常见的恶性肿瘤,也是导致癌症相关死亡的一大重要原因[1]。手术是胃肠道恶性肿瘤根治的唯一治疗选择,然而由于缺乏特异性的临床症状,导致通常的延迟诊断,出现无法治愈的晚期疾病[2]。由于破坏性增殖的肿瘤细胞代谢过程不断增加,进而导致肿瘤微环境中供氧应不足,乏氧已被认为是恶性肿瘤标志之一[3-4]。乏氧可能导致细胞获得更具攻击性的表型[5],被认为是肿瘤转移和血管生成的危险因素之一[6-7]。同时,肿瘤组织的乏氧微环境又会降低肿瘤组织对于常规放化疗以及光疗等各种疗法的敏感性[8-10],是肿瘤治疗成功的主要障碍之一[11-13]。

光动力治疗(Photodynamics Therapy, PDT)是一种新兴的很有前景的肿瘤治疗方式,其主要机制是在激光照射下,激发光敏剂与邻近氧分子之间的能量转移,进而产生大量的活性氧(Reactive Oxygen Species, ROS)来杀死肿瘤细胞[14-16]。由于光动力治疗需要消耗氧气,所以其疗效随着治疗期间氧气的消耗呈指数下降,因此,持续的氧气供应就显得尤为重要[17-22]。到目前为止,已经有不同的策略来克服肿瘤局部乏氧所带来的治疗相关的一系列问题,从而提高PDT的疗效,例如通过全氟化碳纳米颗粒输送额外的氧气,通过吸入提供高压氧等[23-25]。在这些方法中,利用纳米材料作为催化剂原位生成氧气是一种非常有效的方式。其中,氧化锰及其相关纳米复合材料可通过催化内源性过氧化氢(H_2O_2)分解生成氧气,改善肿瘤乏氧问题,近年来备受关注[26-28]。

线粒体作为细胞呼吸过程中不可缺少的细胞器,在人类各种疾病,特别是恶性肿瘤中发挥着重要作用[29-30]。同时,线粒体中大量ROS的堆积会导致线粒体功能障碍,引起细胞凋亡途径,也被认为是癌症治疗中的主要凋亡方式[31-33]。因此,将线粒体作为光动力治疗时的靶细胞器,使光敏剂定位在线粒体内,之后产生的ROS也会在线粒体内积聚,达到很好的治疗效果[34-35]。近红外(Near-Infrared, NIR)光敏剂IR780(图2-1)是一种亲脂阳离子,由于肿瘤细胞的线粒体膜电位较高而主要蓄积在肿瘤细胞的线粒体中[36]。由于线粒体对ROS的脆弱性,IR780介导的线粒体靶向PDT能迅速破坏细胞器的生物学功能,导致肿瘤细胞的凋亡[37-38]。同时,IR780作为一种NIR光敏剂,可以准确地检测肿瘤的位置。

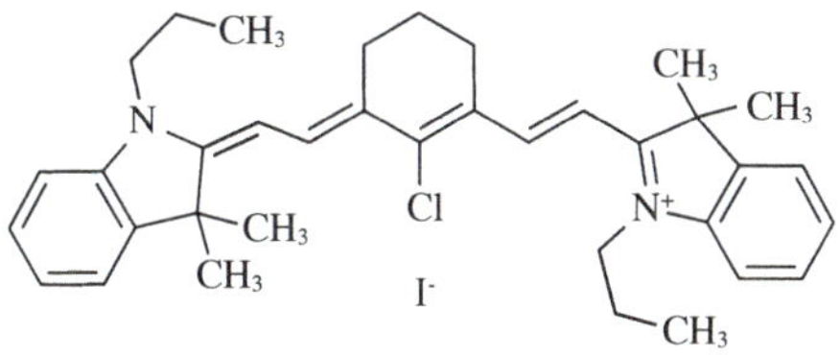

第 2 章 构建线粒体靶向型产氧纳米颗粒实现胃肠道恶性肿瘤的靶向诊断及增强的光动力治疗

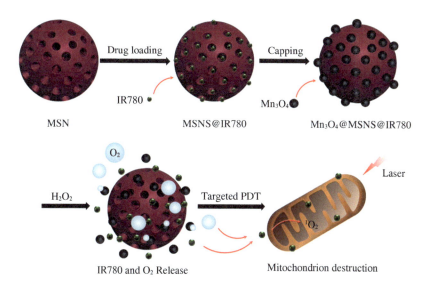

图 2-1 IR780 的分子结构

图 2-2 Mn_3O_4@MSNs@IR780 的合成过程、Mn_3O_4 分解 H_2O_2 释放 IR780 并产生 O_2 以及线粒体靶向的 PDT 治疗过程示意图

图片来自参考文献[48]

基于以上设计,设计合成了一种可同时实现胃肠道恶性肿瘤近红外诊断、氧释放、线粒体靶向药物递送的增强光动力学治疗的一种诊疗一体化的多功能纳米复合材料(Mn_3O_4@MSNs@IR780)。如图 2-2 所示,四氧化三锰(Mn_3O_4)作为门卫,阻挡加载了疏水性光敏剂 IR780 的多孔硅(MSNs)通道。H_2O_2 是肿瘤代谢物之一(大量存在,最高可达 1 mM),本节中的 Mn_3O_4 是一种有效的催化剂,可在无外部活化的情况下持续将 H_2O_2 分解为氧气[39-41]。此外,Mn_3O_4 在分解 H_2O_2 的同时会崩解,暴露出被其封闭的通道。之后,IR780 在肿瘤组织中释放,由于其独特的特性,进而特异性地堆积在肿瘤细胞的线粒体内。在氧气和 808 nm 激光照射的协同作用下,IR780 产生 ROS 损伤线粒体,导致肿瘤细胞凋亡。这种自产氧联合线粒体靶向的光动力治疗可能为扩大 PDT 疗效开辟新途径。

2.2 材料与方法

2.2.1 实验材料与仪器

1) 主要实验材料

胎牛血清(Fetal Bovine Serum,FBS)、RPMI-1640 细胞培养基、无酚红 RPMI-1640 细胞培养基、胰蛋白酶、磷酸盐缓冲溶液(Phosphate Buffered Saline, PBS)、链霉素、青霉素(美国 Gibco);MitoTracker® Green FM 线粒体绿色荧光探针、LysoTracker Green DND-26 溶酶体绿色荧光探针、Calcein-AM/PI 活细胞/死细胞双染试剂盒(中国翊圣);4%多聚甲醛固定液、活性氧检测试剂盒、细胞膜蛋白与细胞浆蛋白提取试剂盒、PVDF 膜、CCK-8 试剂盒(中国碧云天);Rabbit mAb♯5174 抗 GAPDH、Rabbit mAb♯36169 抗 HIF-1α 一抗抗体(美国 Cell Signaling);Pierce 化学发光底物(美国 Thermo Fisher);The Hydrogen Peroxide(H_2O_2) Colorimetric Assay Kit(武汉伊莱瑞特);乙酸锰、N,N-二甲基甲酰胺(DMF)、3-氨丙基三乙氧基硅烷(APTES)、十六烷基三甲基溴化铵(CTAB)、正硅酸乙酯(TEOS)、无水乙醇、琥珀酸酐、三乙胺、二甲基亚砜(Dimethyl Sulfoxide,DMSO)、N-(3-二甲基氨基丙基)-N'-乙基碳二亚胺盐酸盐(EDC·HCl)、IR780(美国 Sigma-Aldrich)。

2) 主要实验仪器

二氧化碳细胞培养箱、-80 ℃实验室超低温冰箱、大容量 ST4 Plus 离心机、ESCALAB-250 X 射线光电子能谱仪(美国 Thermo Fisher);便携式溶解氧测定仪(美国 YSI);Ⅱ类生物安全柜(新加坡 ESCO);玻底培养皿(中国 NEST);纯水仪(美国 Millipore);SX-700 高压蒸汽灭菌锅(日本 TOMY);IX71 荧光倒置显微镜(日本 OLYMPUS);激光共聚焦扫描显微镜(Confocal Laser Scanning Microscope,CLSM)(德国 Leica);SpectraMax iD5-多功能酶标仪(美国 Molecular Devices);LSRFortessa™ 流式细胞分析仪(美国 BD);Maestro™ In-Vivo Imaging System(美国 Cri);Nexus 128 临床前光声计算机断层扫描仪(美国 Endra);透射电子显微镜、高分辨率透射电子显微镜、场发射扫描电子显微镜(日本 JEOL);动态光散射仪(英国 Malvern);ZetaPlus 型 Zeta 电位仪(美国 Brookhaven);荧光光谱仪(日本 HoribaScientific);NexION 300D ICP-MS(美国 PerkinElmer);粉末 X 射线衍射仪(日本 Rigaku);UV-3600 紫外分光光

度计(日本 Shimadzu);Autosorb iQ2 物理吸附仪(美国 Quantachrome)。

2.2.2 实验方法

1) 胺官能化 Mn_3O_4 与羧基官能化 MSNs 的合成

以乙酸锰为原料,采用热分解法制备纳米级 Mn_3O_4。具体来说,将乙酸锰(10 mL)溶解在装有 DMF(50 mL)的烧瓶中,之后将温度提高到 130 ℃。温度稳定后,向上述溶液中加入 APTES(500 μL),生成胺官能化的 Mn_3O_4 纳米级棕色沉淀。最后离心产物,用无水乙醇洗涤三次即可得到。

采用以下方法合成了羧基官能化 MSNs。首先将 CTAB(0.5 g)溶于水(240 mL)中,然后将浓度为 2 mol/L 的氢氧化钠水溶液(1.7 mL)加入上述溶液,并使混合物的温度升高至 80 ℃。之后将 TEOS(2.5 mL)和 APTES(250 μL)逐滴加入上述碱性表面活性剂溶液中,将混合物搅拌 2 h 以获得白色沉淀。过滤所得固体产物,用水和无水乙醇洗涤三次,并在 60 ℃下干燥。最后使用琥珀酸酐(5 mg)和三乙胺(5 μL)加入 DMSO(10 mL)并加入上述固体产物,进一步将 $MSNs-NH_2$ 羧基官能化,得到羧基官能化的 MSNs。

2) MSNs@IR780 与 Mn_3O_4@MSNs@IR780 的制备

首先将光敏剂 IR780(5 mg/mL 溶于乙醇溶液)超声加载到羧基官能化 MSNs(50 mg)中,室温搅拌 10 h。之后离心得到绿色 MSNs@IR780 粉末,用乙醇和水洗涤三次。通过测定剩余溶液以及洗涤液中 IR780 的量来推算其装载量。

用 EDC 化学方法将胺官能化的 Mn_3O_4 固定在 MSNs@IR780 的表面。具体来说,首先将 EDC·HCl(5 mg)、MSNs@IR780(20 mg)和胺官能化的 Mn_3O_4(100 mg)加入水(5 mL)中,搅拌 30 min。最后离心收集沉淀并洗涤三次,即可得到 Mn_3O_4@MSNs@IR780 多功能纳米复合材料。

3) 形貌与表征

使用透射电子显微镜(Transmission Electron Microscopy,TEM)、高分辨透射电子显微镜、场发射扫描电子显微镜(Scanning Electron Microscopy,SEM)和动态光散射(Dynamic Light Scattering,DLS)研究了纳米复合材料的形貌与尺寸。每隔 12 h,测定 Mn_3O_4@MSNs@IR780 纳米颗粒在 PBS 和血清中 DLS 和 Zeta 电位,观察其稳定性。用 IR780 和 Mn_3O_4@MSNs@IR78 纳米颗粒的荧光特性使用荧光分光光度计进行检测。采用宽/小角 X 射线衍射(X-ray Diffraction,XRD)技术测定其结构表征。氮的吸附/解吸等温线由物理吸附仪在 77 K,即 －196 ℃下收集。X射线光电子能谱(X-ray Photoelectron Spectroscopy,XPS)结果使用光电子能谱测定。使用便携式溶解氧测定仪测量氧气产量。傅里叶变换红外光谱(Fourier Transform Infrared,FTIR)和紫外-可见-近红外(Ultraviolet-visible-Near-Infrared,UV-vis-NIR)光谱结果用于监测 IR780 的装载与释放。

4) 响应性 IR780 释放及产氧能力测定

为了研究 Mn_3O_4@MSNs@IR780 催化过氧化氢产生氧气的能力,使用过氧化氢比色分析试剂盒(405 nm)测定 H_2O_2 的浓度。通过 XPS 谱中 Mn^{2p} 峰的出现,揭示了 Mn_3O_4 在 H_2O_2 中孵育 24 h 后的崩解过程。在将纳米材料加入 H_2O_2 后,用便携式溶解氧仪在溶液中的氧电极探头实时测量氧浓度。采用紫外-可见-近红外光谱法测定 IR780 在 780 nm 处的吸光度,反映其控制释放的性能。通过 ICP 法测定 Mn^{2+} 浓度,研究了 Mn_3O_4@MSNs@IR780 的 H_2O_2 浓度依赖性分解行为。

5) 细胞培养

从中国科学院上海细胞生物学研究所获取人胃癌细胞株 MKN-45P,RPMI-1640 细胞培养基中添加了无菌的 FBS(10%)、青霉素(1%)和链霉素(100 g/mL),培养在 37 ℃、5% CO_2 的环境中。当细胞培养至培养皿面积约 85%时,按照 1∶3 比例进行传代。

6) Mn_3O_4@MSNs@IR780 的亚细胞定位

为了证明其线粒体靶向性,使用线粒体和溶酶体选择性荧光探针作为亚细胞定位标记。将 MKN-45P 细胞与 Mn_3O_4@MSNs@IR780 共培养 4 h 后,分别加入线粒体绿色荧光探针($\lambda_{ex}/\lambda_{em}$＝490 nm/516 nm)和溶酶体绿色荧光探针($\lambda_{ex}/\lambda_{em}$＝504 nm/511 nm)标记线粒体和溶酶体,共培养 45 min。之后用 PBS 洗涤三次,用 CLSM 观察 Mn_3O_4@MSNs@IR780 在细胞中的亚细胞定位。

7) 胃肠道恶性肿瘤细胞内 ROS 的检测

活性氧检测试剂盒($\lambda_{ex}/\lambda_{em}$＝488 nm/525 nm)检测胃肠道恶性肿瘤细胞中 ROS 的生成。共分为对照、激光照射、IR780、IR780＋激光照射、Mn_3O_4@MSNs@IR780、Mn_3O_4@MSNs@IR780＋激光照射 6 组。将 MKN-45P 细胞接

第 2 章 构建线粒体靶向型产氧纳米颗粒实现胃肠道恶性肿瘤的靶向诊断及增强的光动力治疗

种于 6 孔板中培养 12 h,然后在 IR780 和 IR780+激光照射组加入 5 μg IR780,最后两组加入含有 5 μg IR780 的 Mn_3O_4@MSNs@IR780 纳米颗粒。37 ℃下孵育 4 h,然后用 PBS 洗涤三次。随后,向每个孔中加入 1 mL 的活性氧检测试剂,孵育 15 min。接着将细胞洗涤三次,并用 808 nm 激光(1 W·cm^{-2})照射 5 min,将细胞洗涤三次,用无酚红 RPMI-1640 细胞培养基重悬。最后用 CLSM 和流式细胞术观察与定量测量 ROS 的产生。

8) 胃肠道恶性肿瘤细胞内乏氧的检测

采用 Western blot 法检测缺氧诱导因子-1α(Hypoxia Inducible Factor-1α,HIF-1α)在胃肠道恶性肿瘤细胞中的表达。使用细胞膜蛋白与细胞浆蛋白提取试剂盒提取 MKN-45P 细胞中的总蛋白,将样品转移到聚偏氟乙烯(Polyvinylidene Fluoride,PVDF)膜上。之后使用 5% 脱脂乳封闭膜,并在 8 ℃条件下与抗 GAPDH 和抗 HIF-1α 一抗孵育过夜。然后使用抗兔二抗,用 Pierce 化学发光底物使条带出现。最后采集照片,并使用 ImageJ 软件进行分析。

9) 体外抗肿瘤治疗效果

采用细胞计数法(Cell Counting Kit-8,CCK-8)和活死细胞双染色法评价其体外抗肿瘤作用。实验分组和处理方式与第 7)条相同。治疗浓度以 IR780 计算,终浓度为 5 μg/mL。将 MKN-45P 细胞接种于 96 孔板中 12 h。37 ℃下孵育 4 h,然后用 PBS 洗涤三次。用 808 nm 激光(1 W·cm^{-2})照射 5 min,将细胞洗涤三次。之后,按照试剂商的说明,在 MKN-45P 细胞悬液中加入 100 μL 双染色检测工作液。共培养 30 min 后,使用 PBS 清洗细胞三次。最后,用激光共焦显微镜观察染色后的活细胞($\lambda_{ex}/\lambda_{em}$=490 nm/515 nm)和死细胞($\lambda_{ex}/\lambda_{em}$=535 nm/617 nm)。至于 CCK-8 法,将 10 μL 试剂加入培养孔中继续共培养 4 h,按照制造商的说明,使用酶标仪在 450 nm 处测量每个孔中的吸光度值。根据说明书指示计算不同处理下的细胞数量。

10) 胃肠道恶性肿瘤异位移植瘤模型的建立

从南京大学模式动物研究所购得 5 周龄重症联合免疫缺陷(Severe Combined Immunodeficiency,SCID)雄性 BALB/c 裸鼠。所有动物实验均经南京大学动物保护与利用委员会(Institutional Animal Care and Use Committee,IACUC)批准,并严格遵守《南京大学实验动物保护与利用指南》。为建立胃肠道恶性肿瘤异位移植瘤模型,将 MKN-45P(1 × 10^6 个)细胞悬浮于 PBS(100 μL)中,皮下注射于裸鼠左腿侧,肿瘤体积按[π/6×长×(宽)^2] 计算。

11) 体内近红外荧光成像与生物分布

将 Mn_3O_4@MSNs@IR780 纳米颗粒溶解于无菌 PBS 中,通过尾静脉注射入胃肠道恶性肿瘤异位移植瘤小鼠体内,浓度为每只小鼠 25 μg/kg 的 IR780。注射后 0 h、0.5 h、1 h、2 h、4 h、6 h、8 h、12 h、24 h、48 h 用 Maestro 活体荧光成像系统对这些小鼠进行成像。在 24 h 麻醉处死小鼠,获得主要器官(心、肝、脾、肺和肾)和肿瘤组织进行离体成像。同时,在尾静脉注射 4 h、12 h、24 h、48 h 后麻醉处死小鼠。收集肿瘤组织和主要器官,称重并在王水中溶解。使用电感耦合等离子体质谱(Inductively Coupled Plasma Mass Spectrometry,ICP-MS)测定其中锰的含量,进而推算纳米粒子的体内生物分布。

12) 体内肿瘤乏氧状态的监测

为监测肿瘤乏氧状态,将异种移植小鼠分为对照、激光照射、IR780、IR780+激光照射、Mn_3O_4@MSNs@IR780、Mn_3O_4@MSNs@IR780+激光照射 6 组。所有注射药物以 IR780 为终浓度,浓度为每只小鼠 25 μg/kg。注射后 24 h,用光声成像(Photoacoustic,PA)监测肿瘤组织中的血管饱和氧含量,使用临床前光声计算机断层扫描仪检测肿瘤内氧合血红蛋白(850 nm)和脱氧血红蛋白(700 nm)浓度。随后麻醉处死小鼠,取肿瘤组织进行 HIF-1α 免疫组化分析。用 ImageJ 软件分析 PA 成像强度以及 HIF-1α 蓝/棕细胞比例。

13) 体内抗肿瘤治疗监测

将胃肠道恶性肿瘤异位移植瘤小鼠随机分为与第 12) 条相同的六组,每组起始治疗时肿瘤体积约 50 mm^3。所有注射药物以 IR780 为终浓度,浓度为每只小鼠 25 μg/kg,对照组每只小鼠注射 100 μL 的 PBS。激光照射、IR780+激光照射以及 Mn_3O_4@MSNs@IR780+激光照射组的每只小鼠使用 808 nm 激光(1 W·cm^{-2})照射 5 min。激光照射后每两天观察并记录小鼠体重和肿瘤体积。16 天后麻醉处死小鼠,收集肿瘤组织,用 PBS 洗涤三次,称重并用 4% 多聚甲醛溶液固定。最后,用苏木精-伊红(Hematoxylin and Eosin,H-E)和 TUNEL 染色,进行免疫组织化学分析。

14) Mn_3O_4@MSNs@IR780 的生物安全性分析

收集主要器官(心、肝、脾、肺和肾),用 4% 多聚甲醛溶液固定之后用石蜡包埋。然后,用 H-E 染色,并用光学显微镜检测组织病理学变化。同时,血液学和血生化分析也被用来评价 Mn_3O_4@MSNs@IR780 的体内毒性以及生物相容性。治疗后第 16 天，麻醉处死小鼠，采集血液进行血液学和血生化检测，包括白细胞(White Blood Cell, WBC)、中性粒细胞(Neutrophil, NEU)、淋巴细胞(Lymphocyte, LYM)、红细胞(Red Blood Cell, RBC)、血红蛋白(Hemoglobin, HGB)、血小板(Platelet, PLT)、谷丙转氨酶(Alanine Aminotransferase, ALT)、谷草转氨酶(Aspartate Aminotransferase, AST)、血尿素氮(Blood Urea Nitrogen, BUN)和血肌酐(Serum creatinine, Scr)。

15) 统计分析

所有数据均使用 GraphPad Prism(5.01 版)软件进行分析，显著性水平为：$*p<0.05$；$**p<0.01$；$***p<0.001$。所有数据均以平均值±标准差(Standard Deviation, SD)表示。

2.3 结果与讨论

2.3.1 Mn_3O_4@MSNs@IR780 的合成与表征

首先合成了以 MSNs 为基础的药物纳米载体，对其羧基功能化修饰，提高了其水稳定性，并为门卫提供了锚定位点。通过超声将 IR780 装载到功能化 MSNs 中，利用 EDC 化学法将直径约 5 nm 的 Mn_3O_4(图 2-3(a))固定在 MSNs(MSNs@IR780)上作为门卫。如扫描电子显微镜(图 2-3(b))和透射电子显微镜(图 2-3(c))图像显示 Mn_3O_4 对 IR780 分子表现出了很强的阻断作用，可以防止 IR780 在到达肿瘤区域之前从 MSNs 的纳米通道泄漏。

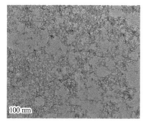
(a) Mn_3O_4 的 TEM 结果图，标尺是 100 nm

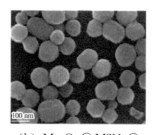
(b) Mn_3O_4@MSNs@IR780 的 SEM 结果图，标尺是 100 nm

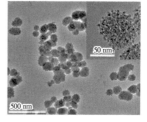
(c) Mn_3O_4@MSNs@IR780 的 TEM 结果图，标尺是 500 nm

图 2-3 纳米粒的形貌特点

图片来自参考文献[48]

在高分辨率 TEM 中可以看到 MSNs 中存在纳米孔(图 2-4(a))。MSNs

的尺寸约为 88 nm，Mn_3O_4@MSNs@IR780 的尺寸约为 94 nm（图 2-4(b)）。Mn_3O_4、MSNs、MSNs@IR780 和 Mn_3O_4@MSNs@IR780 的 Zeta 电位分别约为 35 mV，-31 mV，-27 mV 和 3 mV（图 2-4(c)），证明 Mn_3O_4 与 MSNs@IR780 表面共轭成功。在加载 IR780 并且与 Mn_3O_4 共轭后，小角 X 射线衍射结果中典型的 MSNs 峰（图 2-4(d)红色箭头所示）显著降低，同时根据氮吸附/解吸等温线所示，在药物装载和表面覆盖后，MSNs 的比表面积也减少很多（图 2-4(e)），共同表明其表面的孔洞已经被 IR780 和 Mn_3O_4 覆盖。根据氮吸附/解吸等温线，计算了三种样品的孔径分布。如图 2-4(f)所示，MSNs 的孔径在约 2.45 nm 处具有窄分布，而在装载后的样品中在 1.4～2.7 nm 处呈宽分布，也证明了 MSNs 的纳米载药通道被成功封堵。同时，Mn_3O_4@MSNs@IR780 的 UV-vis-NIR（图 2-4(g)）以及 FTIR（图 2-4(h)）光谱结果均具有 IR780 和 Mn_3O_4 的特定吸收峰，可证明疏水光敏剂和 H_2O_2 响应开关的成功加载。

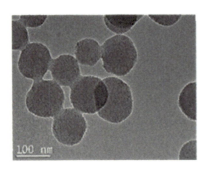

(a) MSNs 的高分辨率透射电镜显微照片，标尺是 100 nm

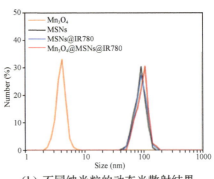

(b) 不同纳米粒的动态光散射结果

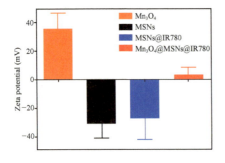

(c) 不同纳米粒的 Zeta 电位结果

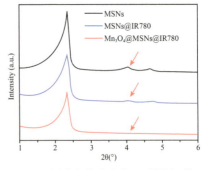

(d) 不同纳米粒的小角 X 射线衍射结果

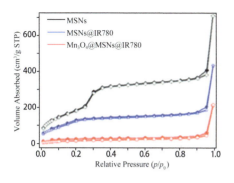
（e）不同纳米粒的氮吸附/解吸等温线

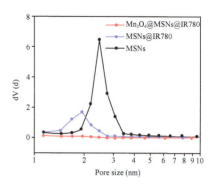
（f）不同纳米粒的相应孔径分布结果

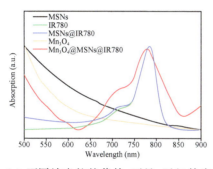
（g）不同纳米粒的紫外-可见-近红外光谱结果

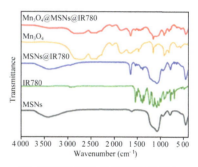
（h）不同纳米粒的傅里叶变换红外光谱结果。数据以平均值±标准差表示

图 2-4 纳米粒的表征结果

图片来自参考文献[48]

2.3.2 $Mn_3O_4@MSNs@IR780$ 的稳定性

如图 2-5(a)所示，IR780 和 $Mn_3O_4@MSNs@IR780$ 纳米颗粒的荧光曲线相似，表明加载到 MSNs 后荧光不会淬灭。同时，$Mn_3O_4@MSNs@IR780$ 纳米颗粒的 DLS(图 2-5(b))和 Zeta 电位(图 2-5(c))结果在 PBS 和血清中能保持 96 h 的稳定，表明其具有良好的稳定性。

2.3.3 纳米颗粒体外 H_2O_2 分解及响应性 IR780 释放

当暴露于肿瘤微环境中特有的高浓度 H_2O_2 时，Mn_3O_4 会迅速溶解，并产生氧气[42-43]。TEM 图像（图 2-6(a)）显示纳米颗粒变得更光滑，表面黑点（Mn_3O_4）更少，也验证这一过程。同时，如宽角 X 射线衍射测试(图 2-6(b))所示,在过氧化氢溶液中,Mn_3O_4 的特征峰显著降低,表明了 Mn_3O_4 的分解和脱落。由氮吸附/解吸等温线结果可知(图 2-6(c)),加入 H_2O_2 中 24 h 后,其比表面积增加很多,同时 FTIR(图 2-6(d))以及 UV-vis-NIR(图 2-6(e))的光谱结果中,可见 IR780 和 Mn_3O_4 的特定吸收峰消失,证明了 Mn_3O_4 的分解脱落以及 IR780 的释放。上述结果表明,Mn_3O_4 被分解,进而打开了 MSNs 的通道。之后,研究了纳米颗粒对于 H_2O_2 的分解效率。如图 2-6(f)所示,Mn_3O_4 和 Mn_3O_4@MSNs @IR780 均可在 3 h 内分解大部分 H_2O_2,表现出相似的分解效率。之后,在过氧化氢中加入不同的纳米粒,使用便携式溶解氧计来确定产生氧气能力,由图 2-6(g)可见,在加入 Mn_3O_4 和 Mn_3O_4@MSNs@IR780 后,实时氧浓度迅速增加,而 MSNs@IR780 几乎没有生成氧气的能力。最后,通过 UV-vis-NIR 监测 IR780 的浓度,验证其释放能力。如图 2-6(h)所示,在 PBS 情况下,Mn_3O_4@MSNs@IR780 纳米粒子中的 IR780 在 12 h 释放了不到 9%,而未使用 Mn_3O_4 封闭的纳米粒子中的 IR780 在 6 h 内的释放量为 35%。当加入 H_2O_2 后,纳米粒子中的 IR780 可以在 6 h 内快速释放。以上结果表明,这种多功能 Mn_3O_4@MSNs @IR780 纳米粒子能够响应富含 H_2O_2 的肿瘤微环境,显著提高氧浓度,并成功释放药物。

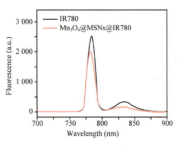

(a) IR780 和 Mn_3O_4@MSNs@IR780 纳米颗粒的荧光光谱

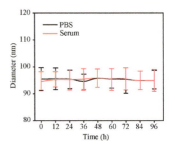

(b) Mn_3O_4@MSNs@IR780 纳米颗粒在 PBS 和血清中每 12 h 的 DLS 结果

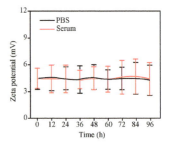

(c) Mn_3O_4@MSNs@IR780 纳米颗粒在 PBS 和血清中每 12 h 的 Zeta 电位结果

数据以平均值±标准差表示。

图 2-5 纳米粒的稳定性

图片来自参考文献[48]

第 2 章 构建线粒体靶向型产氧纳米颗粒实现胃肠道恶性肿瘤的靶向诊断及增强的光动力治疗

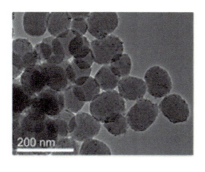

（a）加入 H_2O_2 后的 TEM 图像

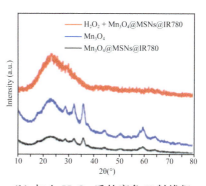

（b）加入 H_2O_2 后的宽角 X 射线衍射结果

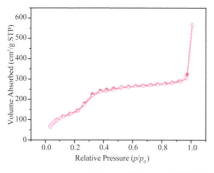

（c）加入 H_2O_2 后的氮吸附/解吸等温线

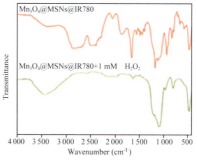

（d）加入 H_2O_2 前后的 FTIR 光谱结果

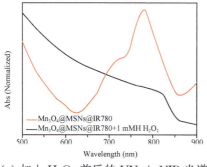

（e）加入 H_2O_2 前后的 UV-vis-NIR 光谱结果

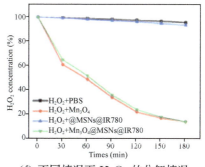

（f）不同情况下 H_2O_2 的分解情况

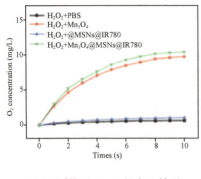 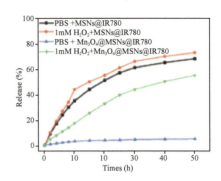

(g) 不同情况下 O_2 的产生情况　　　(h) IR780 在不同模拟条件下的释放曲线

图 2-6　Mn_3O_4@MSNs@IR780 纳米颗粒体外 H_2O_2 分解及响应性 IR780 释放

图片来自参考文献[48]

2.3.4　Mn_3O_4@MSNs@IR780 纳米颗粒的亚细胞定位

作为一种亲脂阳离子,由于肿瘤细胞中线粒体膜电位较高,IR780 可在细胞内与线粒体特异性结合[44-45]。为了验证 Mn_3O_4@MSNs@IR780 可在肿瘤细胞内特异性靶向线粒体,进而发挥高效的 PDT 能力,我们比较了其和线粒体/溶酶体定位探针的亚细胞定位。如图 2-7(a)所示,Mn_3O_4@MSNs@IR780 的红色信号定位与线粒体的绿色荧光极为相似,而与溶酶体的绿色荧光不相似。对 CLSM 结果进行共定位分析,溶酶体(图 2-7(b))和线粒体(图 2-7(c))均可得到相似的结果。以上结果表明在 MKN-45P 细胞中,Mn_3O_4@MSNs@IR780 纳米颗粒可以特异性地靶向线粒体。

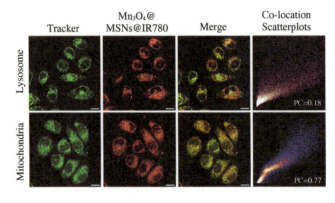

(a) 使用激光共聚焦及线粒体/溶酶体定位探针(绿色)来展示纳米颗粒的亚细胞定位,标尺是 10 μm

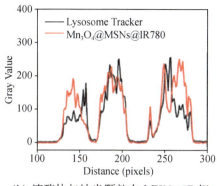
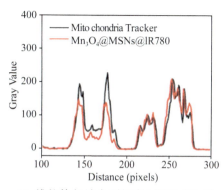

(b) 溶酶体与纳米颗粒在 MKN-45P 细胞中的共定位分析

(c) 线粒体与纳米颗粒在 MKN-45P 细胞中的共聚焦分析

图 2-7　Mn_3O_4@MSNs@IR780 的亚细胞定位

图片来自参考文献[48]

2.3.5　胃肠道恶性肿瘤细胞中乏氧的检测

接下来的研究是为了证明 Mn_3O_4@MSNs@IR780 产生氧气可以抑制乏氧相关的信号通路。蛋白印迹结果(图 2-8(a))显示，对照、激光照射和 IR780 组细胞上清的 HIF-1α 表达相似，无统计学差异。而 IR780+激光照射组 HIF-1α 蛋白水平明显高于其他所有组，表明 PDT 单独治疗可导致癌细胞中乏氧环境的加剧。相比之下，Mn_3O_4@MSNs@IR780+激光照射组的 HIF-1α 水平最低。定量分析结果(图 2-8(b))也证明了以上结论，表明 Mn_3O_4@MSNs@IR780 可以通过释放氧气，抑制乏氧相关的信号通路，进而改善肿瘤乏氧微环境，达到增强 PDT 的作用。

2.3.6　胃肠道恶性肿瘤细胞中 ROS 产量的检测

由于 ROS 具有很高的细胞毒性，因此能直接杀死肿瘤细胞[46-47]。为检测在 808 nm 的激光照射下，这种纳米颗粒是否能在细胞内产生 ROS，将 IR780 和 Mn_3O_4@MSNs@IR780 与 MKN-45P 细胞共培养，使用 DCFH-DA 检测 ROS 的生成情况。如图 2-9(a)所示，经过 808 nm 激光($1\ W\cdot cm^{-2}$)照射 5 min 后，Mn_3O_4@MSNs@IR780+激光照射组显示出了最高的绿色荧光，表明产生了 ROS。同时，在 IR780+激光照射组可观察到少量绿色荧光，表明纳米颗粒可以有效地增加细胞内 ROS 的生成。之后，利用流式细胞术进一步定量分析活性氧的产生情况。图 2-9(b)展现出了类似的结果，即 Mn_3O_4@MSNs@

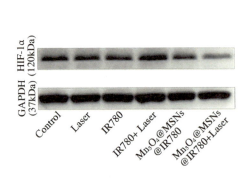
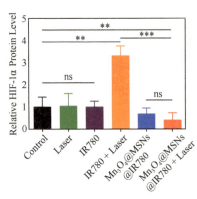

(a) Western blot 检测细胞上清液中 HIF-1α 蛋白水平

(b) 定量分析 Western blot 结果

数据以平均值±标准差表示,ns 代表没有统计学差异,** 代表 $p<0.01$；*** 代表 $p<0.001$。

图 2-8　不同处理后胃肠道恶性肿瘤细胞中乏氧的检测

图片来自参考文献[48]

IR780＋激光照射组荧光强度最高,定量分析表明存在显著统计学差异(*** $p<0.001$,图 2-9(c))。以上结果证实,在激光照射下,Mn_3O_4@MSNs@IR780 由于可以在肿瘤局部产生氧气,可以比 IR780 产生更多的 ROS,进而达到更好的 PDT 疗效。

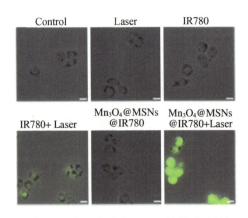

(a) 细胞中 ROS 产量检测的 CLSM 结果,标尺是 20 μm

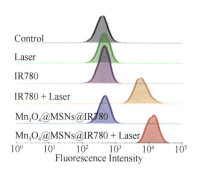
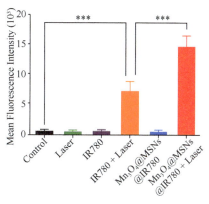

(b) 细胞中 ROS 产量检测的流式细胞术结果

(c) 定量分析流式细胞术结果

数据以平均值±标准差表示，***代表 $p < 0.001$。

图 2-9 不同处理后 MKN-45P 细胞中 ROS 产量的检测

图片来自参考文献[48]

2.3.7 Mn$_3$O$_4$@MSNs@IR780 的体外抗肿瘤治疗效果

在检测 Mn$_3$O$_4$@MSNs@IR780 的产氧、产生 ROS 和线粒体靶向能力后，使用 Calcein-AM/PI 和 CCK-8 方法评价其对于 MKN-45P 细胞的杀伤作用。如图 2-10(a)所示，对照组未见明显红色细胞，激光照射、IR780 和 Mn$_3$O$_4$@MSNs@IR780 可见少量的红色细胞。在 IR780+激光照射组，可观察到中等数量的 MKN-45P 细胞呈红色，说明 IR780 对于胃肠道恶性肿瘤细胞存在一定的杀伤作用。而在 Mn$_3$O$_4$@MSNs@IR780+激光照射组中，几乎所有的 MKN-45P 细胞都发出红色荧光，基本没有可见的绿色细胞。使用 ImageJ 定量分析绿色细胞比例，可得到相同的结果(图 2-10(b))。之后，使用 CCK-8 法进一步检测不同组细胞的活力。如图 2-10(c)所示，当 IR780 浓度固定(5 μg/mL)时，引入 Mn$_3$O$_4$@MSNs 可显著提升 IR780 的体外光动力治疗效果。以上结果表明，这种纳米颗粒在体外具有较好的生物安全性，同时在 808 nm 激光的照射下，对于 MKN-45P 细胞具有较强的光动力治疗作用，可进一步用于体内的肿瘤治疗。

2.3.8 活体近红外荧光成像与体内生物分布

体外研究后，采用胃肠道恶性肿瘤异位移植瘤模型进行体内实验。第一步，需要确定纳米颗粒在体内的分布情况，选择最合适的给药后时间点进行激

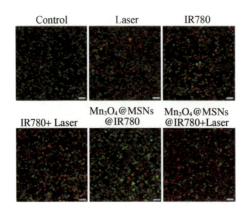

(a) 使用 Calcein-AM/PI 活死细胞双染试剂盒拍摄不同处理后细胞的 CLSM 图像。绿色荧光表示活细胞,红色荧光表示死细胞,标尺是 50 μm

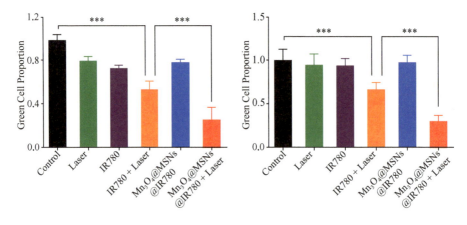

(b) 绿色细胞数占总细胞数的比例

(c) 使用 CCK-8 试剂盒测定不同处理后的细胞活力

数据以平均值±标准差表示,** 代表 $p<0.01$;*** 代表 $p<0.001$。

图 2-10　不同处理后细胞毒性的检测

图片来自参考文献[48]

光照射。首先,尾静脉注射 Mn_3O_4@MSNs@IR780 纳米颗粒后,使用实时活体荧光成像系统在不同时间点采集实时近红外成像结果。用不同的颜色显示不同的荧光强度,荧光强度按红、黄、绿、蓝的顺序递减。如图 2-11(a)所示,荧光信号在注射后 4 h 可在肿瘤区域观察到,注射后 24 h 在肿瘤组织中检测到最强的荧光信号。尾静脉注射 24 h 后心、肝、脾、肺、肾和肿瘤组织的离体近红外荧光也证明了肿瘤组织具有很强烈的荧光(图 2-11(b))。肿瘤的活体(图 2-11

(c))及离体(图2-11(d))荧光强度结果也证明了纳米颗粒在注射后0.5 h开始在肿瘤组织积累,并且在24 h达到峰值。如图2-11(e)所示,根据锰含量的ICP-MS结果,Mn_3O_4@MSNs@IR780纳米颗粒在肝组织中积累最多。同时,肿瘤组织中的锰浓度在尾静脉注射后24小时达到峰值,显示出与活体近红外荧光成像相同的结果。以上结果可以证明,Mn_3O_4@MSNs@IR780纳米颗粒在体内主要经由肝脏代谢,并且可通过实体瘤的高通透性和滞留(Enhanced Permeability and Retention,EPR)效应,特异性地在体内靶向肿瘤组织,进而降低对其他器官的非特异性毒性,并且发挥胃肠道恶性肿瘤诊断与治疗相结合的效果。

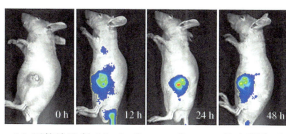

(a) 尾静脉注射 Mn_3O_4@MSNs@IR780 纳米颗粒后不同时间点胃肠道恶性肿瘤异位移植瘤小鼠的实时活体近红外荧光图像

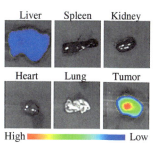

(b) 尾静脉注射 24 h 后心、肝、脾、肺、肾和肿瘤组织的离体近红外荧光

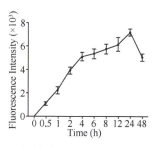

(c) 尾静脉注射后不同时间点肿瘤的活体荧光信号强度

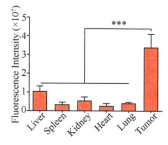

(d) 心、肝、脾、肺、肾和肿瘤组织的离体荧光信号强度

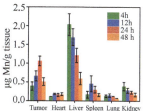

(e) 根据锰浓度推算尾静脉注射纳米颗粒后不同时间点的体内生物分布

数据以平均值±标准差表示,*** 代表 $p<0.001$。

图2-11 Mn_3O_4@MSNs@IR780 的活体近红外荧光成像与体内生物分布

图片来自参考文献[48]

2.3.9 体内胃肠道恶性肿瘤组织乏氧情况的监测

进一步检测 Mn_3O_4@MSNs@IR780 治疗是否可以改善肿瘤组织的乏氧状况。首先,使用光声成像检测尾静脉注射 24 h 后小鼠肿瘤组织的氧合血红蛋白及脱氧血红蛋白情况,实时监测肿瘤组织的含氧情况。由图 2-12(a)可知,注射后 24 h,Mn_3O_4@MSNs@IR780+激光照射组氧合血红蛋白含量最高,脱氧血红蛋白最低。相应地,IR780+激光照射组的结果正好相反。其余四组之间并没有明显差异(图 2-12(c)、图 2-12(d))。这些结果表明,这种纳米颗粒可以成功地在小鼠体内增加局部氧供,进而改善肿瘤乏氧。之后,收集小鼠的肿瘤组织进行 HIF-1α 免疫组化染色,判断乏氧相关信号通路是否受到抑制(图 2-12(b))。由图 2-12(e)可知,IR780+激光照射组的 HIF-1α 水平最高,显著高于其他五组。同时,Mn_3O_4@MSNs@IR780+激光照射组的 HIF-1α 水平与对照组相比并无显著性差异。以上结果证明了该疗法能有效增加局部氧供,抑制肿瘤乏氧微环境,进而抑制 MKN-45P 细胞的乏氧信号通路。

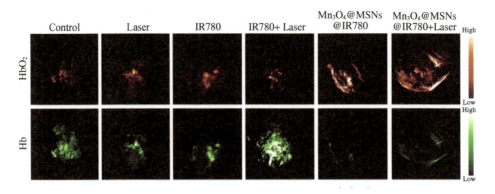

(a) 尾静脉注射 24 h 后肿瘤组织的光声成像

使用氧合血红蛋白(HbO_2)和脱氧血红蛋白(Hb)联合实时监测肿瘤组织的含氧情况。

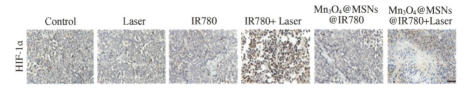

(b) 尾静脉注射 24 h 后 HIF-1α 免疫组织化学染色结果

蓝色为 HIF-1α 阴性细胞,棕色为 HIF-1α 阳性细胞,标尺是 50 μm。

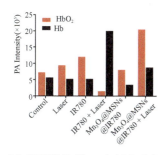
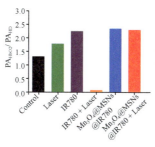
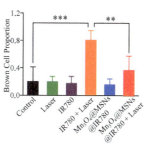

(c) 尾静脉注射 24 h 氧合血红蛋白和脱氧血红蛋白的 PA 强度

(d) 氧合血红蛋白与脱氧血红蛋白强度之比

(e) HIF-1α 免疫组织化学结果中棕色细胞数占总细胞数的比例

数据以平均值±标准差表示，** 代表 $p < 0.01$；*** 代表 $p < 0.001$。

图 2-12 不同处理后肿瘤乏氧状态的检测

图片来自参考文献[48]

2.3.10 体内抗肿瘤治疗效果

之前结果表明，在 808 nm 激光照射下，Mn_3O_4@MSNs@IR780 有效地杀伤 MKN-45P 细胞，也可改善小鼠体内乏氧微环境，因此进一步观察了其体内抗肿瘤作用。由前活体近红外成像和生物分布结果，选择为静脉注射后 24 h 为 808 nm 激光的照射时间点。最终的治疗浓度为每只小鼠 25 μg/kg 的 IR780。如图 2-13(a)所示，对照、激光照射、IR780 和 Mn_3O_4@MSNs@IR780 组肿瘤生长迅速，未达到有效的治疗效果。IR780 组的肿瘤前四天生长缓慢。然而，四天后肿瘤速度明显加快，也未取得较好的治疗效果。相比之下，Mn_3O_4@MSNs@IR780+激光照射组中肿瘤体积几乎没有增加，表现出了显著增强的治疗效果。肿瘤照片(图 2-13(b))和肿瘤重量(图 2-13(c))也显示出了相似的趋势。肿瘤组织切片的 H-E 和 TUNEL 染色结果(图 2-13(d))也可在 Mn_3O_4@MSNs@IR780+激光照射组观察到最多的细胞坏死与凋亡。因此，我们推测肿瘤乏氧可能会持续抑制光动力治疗的效果，导致肿瘤复发和不良预后。而这种多功能纳米颗粒能显著改善肿瘤乏氧微环境，进而增强 PDT 对肿瘤生长和复发的抑制作用。

2.3.11 生物安全分析

为了评估纳米颗粒的体内生物安全性，在不同的治疗的过程中，监测小鼠体重，期间几乎没有发现体重存在波动(图 2-14(a))。同时，结束后收集了小鼠

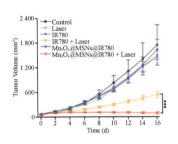
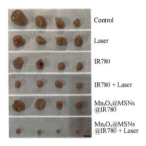
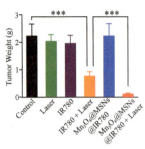

(a) 治疗 16 天的肿瘤生长曲线　　(b) 治疗 16 天后的肿瘤照片　　(c) 治疗 16 天后的肿瘤重量

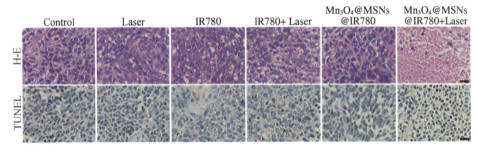

(d) 治疗 16 天后肿瘤组织的 H-E 和 TUNEL 染色结果，标尺是 50 μm

数据以平均值±标准差表示，*** 代表 $p<0.001$。

图 2-13　不同治疗后体内抗肿瘤治疗效果检测

图片来自参考文献[48]

血液进行血生化(图 2-14(b))和血液学(图 2-14(c))分析，评估其潜在细胞毒性。各组的肝功能(ALT、AST)、肾功能(BUN、Scr)、免疫应答反应(WBC、NEU、LYM)、细胞毒性(RBC、HGB)和脾功能(PLT)结果均未存在显著性差异。最后，收集小鼠的心、肝、脾、肺和肾进行 H-E 染色。如图 2-14(d)所示，所有组均表现出可忽略的炎症损伤、组织学异常以及坏死。以上结果表明这种多功能纳米颗粒 Mn_3O_4@MSNs@IR780 治疗时具有很高的生物安全性，主要原因可能是由于肿瘤靶向给药以及肿瘤微环境的控制释放，降低了对非肿瘤器官的副作用。

2.4　总结

本节成功地制备了可同时实现胃肠道恶性肿瘤近红外诊断、氧释放、线粒体

第 2 章 构建线粒体靶向型产氧纳米颗粒实现胃肠道恶性肿瘤的靶向诊断及增强的光动力治疗

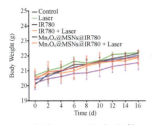

(a) 治疗 16 天的小鼠体重曲线

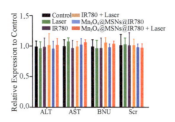

(b) 治疗 16 天后的血清生化检查,包括谷丙转氨酶(ALT)、谷草转氨酶(AST)、血尿素氮(BUN)和血肌酐(Scr)

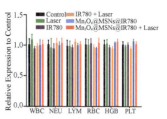

(c) 治疗 16 天后的血液学检查,包括白细胞(WBC)、中性粒细胞(NEU)、淋巴细胞(LYM)、红细胞(RBC)、血红蛋白(HGB)和血小板(PLT)

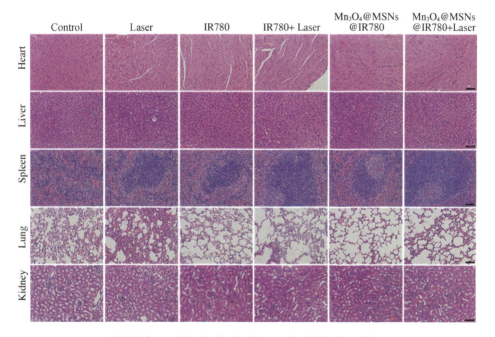

(d) 主要器官(心、肝、脾、肺、肾)的 H-E 切片染色,标尺是 50 μm

数据以平均值±标准差表示。

图 2-14　不同治疗后体内生物安全性分析

图片来自参考文献[48]

靶向药物递送增强光动力学治疗的 Mn_3O_4@MSNs@IR780 这种诊疗一体化的多功能纳米复合材料。体外研究表明,Mn_3O_4 在富含 H_2O_2 的肿瘤微环境中,

可分解 H_2O_2 并持续产生氧气。在 H_2O_2 分解过程中，Mn_3O_4 作为多孔硅通道的"门卫"也溶解、脱落，从而使其内部 IR780 得以释放。随后，释放的 IR780 进一步特异性地靶向胃肠道恶性肿瘤细胞的线粒体并在激光照射下产生 ROS，破坏其生物功能，从而促进细胞的凋亡和坏死。氧气的产生可以减轻乏氧肿瘤微环境，如体内光声成像所示。肿瘤乏氧的清除也被证实能增强光动力治疗的效果并防止肿瘤复发，进而获得良好的预后。总之，本部分证实了一种通过氧补充来克服传统治疗中的乏氧限制并且靶向线粒体来增强光动力治疗的破坏能力的新方法，或为胃肠道恶性肿瘤的纳米诊断治疗一体化提供一些帮助[48]。

参考文献

[1] SEIDLITZ T, MERKER S R, ROTHE A, et al. Human gastric cancer modelling using organoids. Gut, 2019, 68(2):207-217.

[2] HUNT R H, CAMILLERI M, CROWE S E, et al. The stomach in health and disease. Gut, 2015, 64(10):1650-1668.

[3] FENG L, CHENG L, DONG Z, et al. Theranostic liposomes with hypoxia-activated prodrug to effectively destruct hypoxic tumors post-photodynamic therapy. ACS Nano, 2017, 11(1):927-937.

[4] JAHANBAN-ESFAHLAN R, DE LA GUARDIA M, AHMADI D, et al. Modulating tumor hypoxia by nanomedicine for effective cancer therapy. J Cell Physiol., 2018, 233(3):2019-2031.

[5] HE C, WANG L, ZHANG J, et al. Hypoxia-inducible microRNA-224 promotes the cell growth, migration and invasion by directly targeting RASSF8 in gastric cancer. Mol Cancer., 2017, 16(1):35.

[6] GILKES D M, SEMENZA G L, WIRTZ D. Hypoxia and the extracellular matrix: drivers of tumour metastasis. Nat Rev Cancer., 2014, 14(6):430-439.

[7] HSU Y L, HUNG J Y, CHANG W A, et al. Hypoxic lung cancer-secreted exosomal miR-23a increased angiogenesis and vascular permeability by targeting prolyl hydroxylase and tight junction protein ZO-1. Oncogene, 2017, 36(34):4929-4942.

[8] SEMENZA G L. The hypoxic tumor microenvironment: A driving force for

breast cancer progression. Biochim Biophys Acta. , 2016, 1863(3):382 - 391.

[9] SWARTZ M A, IIDA N, ROBERTS E W, et al. Tumor microenvironment complexity: emerging roles in cancer therapy. Cancer Res. , 2012, 72(10):2473 - 2480.

[10] BARKER H E, PAGET J T, KHAN A A, et al. The tumour microenvironment after radiotherapy: mechanisms of resistance and recurrence. Nat Rev Cancer. , 2015, 15(7):409 - 425.

[11] ZHANG Y, WANG F, LIU C, et al. Nanozyme decorated metal-organic frameworks for enhanced photodynamic therapy. ACS Nano, 2018, 12(1):651 - 661.

[12] SONG X, FENG L, LIANG C, et al. Liposomes co-loaded with metformin and chlorin e6 modulate tumor hypoxia during enhanced photodynamic therapy. Nano Research, 2017, 10(4): 1200 - 1212.

[13] CHENG Y, CHENG H, JIANG C, et al. Perfluorocarbon nanoparticles enhance reactive oxygen levels and tumour growth inhibition in photodynamic therapy. Nat Commun. , 2015, 6:8785.

[14] ZHANG W, LU J, GAO X, et al. Enhanced photodynamic therapy by reduced levels of intracellular glutathione obtained by employing a Nano-MOF with Cu^{II} as the active center. Angew Chem Int Ed Engl. , 2018, 57(18):4891 - 4896.

[15] TSAI W H, YU K H, HUANG Y C, et al. EGFR-targeted photodynamic therapy by curcumin-encapsulated chitosan/TPP nanoparticles. Int J Nanomedicine. , 2018, 13:903 - 916.

[16] PAN W, SHI M, LI Y, et al. A GSH-responsive nanophotosensitizer for efficient photodynamic therapy. RSC Adv. , 2018, 8(74):42374 - 42379.

[17] SONG M, LIU T, SHI C, et al. Bioconjugated manganese dioxide nanoparticles enhance chemotherapy response by priming tumor-associated macrophages toward M1-like phenotype and attenuating tumor hypoxia. ACS Nano, 2016, 10(1):633 - 647.

[18] YAO C, WANG W, WANG P, et al. Near-infrared upconversion mesoporous cerium oxide hollow biophotocatalyst for concurrent pH-/H_2O_2-

Responsive O_2-Evolving synergetic cancer therapy. Adv Mater., 2018, 30(7):201704833.

[19] LIU Y, LIU Y, BU W, et al. Hypoxia induced by upconversion-based photodynamic therapy: towards highly effective synergistic bioreductive therapy in tumors. Angew Chem Int Ed Engl., 2015, 54(28):8105-8109.

[20] LIU J, LIANG H, LI M, et al. Tumor acidity activating multifunctional nanoplatform for NIR-mediated multiple enhanced photodynamic and photothermal tumor therapy. Biomaterials, 2018, 157:107-124.

[21] ZHANG M, CUI Z, SONG R, et al. $SnWO_4$-based nanohybrids with full energy transfer for largely enhanced photodynamic therapy and radiotherapy. Biomaterials, 2018, 155:135-144.

[22] KIM J, CHO H R, JEON H, et al. Continuous O_2-Evolving $MnFe_2O_4$ nanoparticle-anchored mesoporous silica nanoparticles for efficient photodynamic therapy in hypoxic cancer. J Am Chem Soc., 2017, 139(32): 10992-10995.

[23] GAO M, LIANG C, SONG X, et al. Erythrocyte-membrane-enveloped perfluorocarbon as nanoscale artificial red blood cells to relieve tumor hypoxia and enhance cancer radiotherapy. Adv Mater., 2017, 29(35):201701429.

[24] ZHANG L, WANG D, YANG K, et al. Mitochondria-targeted artificial "Nano-RBCs" for amplified synergistic cancer phototherapy by a single NIR irradiation. Adv Sci(Weinh)., 2018, 5(8):1800049.

[25] Day R A, Estabrook D A, Logan J K, et al. Fluorous photosensitizers enhance photodynamic therapy with perfluorocarbon nanoemulsions. Chem Commun(Camb)., 2017, 53(97):13043-13046.

[26] CHEN Q, FENG L, LIU J, et al. Intelligent albumin-MnO_2 nanoparticles as pH-/H_2O_2-Responsive dissociable nanocarriers to modulate tumor hypoxia for effective combination therapy. Adv Mater., 2016, 28(33):7129-7136.

[27] Zhu W, Dong Z, Fu T, et al. Modulation of hypoxia in solid tumor microenvironment with MnO_2 nanoparticles to enhance photodynamic therapy. Advanced Functional Materials, 2016, 26(30):5490-5498.

[28] GAO S, WANG G, QIN Z, et al. Oxygen-generating hybrid nanoparticles to enhance fluorescent/photoacoustic/ultrasound imaging guided tumor photodynamic therapy. Biomaterials, 2017, 112: 324 – 335.

[29] LIU S, FENG M, GUAN W. Mitochondrial DNA sensing by STING signaling participates in inflammation, cancer and beyond. Int J Cancer., 2016, 139(4): 736 – 741.

[30] ZHOU W, YU H, ZHANG L J, et al. Redox-triggered activation of nanocarriers for mitochondria-targeting cancer chemotherapy. Nanoscale, 2017, 9(43): 17044 – 17053.

[31] LI N, YU L, WANG J, et al. A mitochondria-targeted nanoradiosensitizer activating reactive oxygen species burst for enhanced radiation therapy. Chem Sci., 2018, 9(12): 3159 – 3164.

[32] LIN M T, BEAL M F. Mitochondrial dysfunction and oxidative stress in neurodegenerative diseases. Nature, 2006, 443(7113): 787 – 795.

[33] KROEMER G, GALLUZZI L, BRENNER C. Mitochondrial membrane permeabilization in cell death. Physiol Rev., 2007, 87(1): 99 – 163.

[34] ZIELONKA J, JOSEPH J, SIKORA A, et al. Mitochondria-targeted triphenylphosphonium-based compounds: syntheses, mechanisms of action, and therapeutic and diagnostic applications. Chem Rev., 2017, 117(15): 10043 – 10120.

[35] JUNG H S, LEE J H, KIM K, et al. A mitochondria-targeted cryptocyanine-based photothermogenic photosensitizer. J Am Chem Soc., 2017, 139(29): 9972 – 9978.

[36] ZHANG C, LIU T, SU Y, et al. A near-infrared fluorescent heptamethine indocyanine dye with preferential tumor accumulation for in vivo imaging. Biomaterials, 2010, 31(25): 6612 – 6617.

[37] MURPHY M P, SMITH R A. Targeting antioxidants to mitochondria byconjugation to lipophilic cations. Annu Rev Pharmacol Toxicol., 2007; 47: 629 – 656.

[38] HORTON K L, STEWART K M, FONSECA S B, et al. Mitochondria-penetrating peptides. Chem Biol., 2008, 15(4): 375 – 382.

[39] REN S, YANG J, MA L, et al. Ternary-responsive drug delivery with activatable dual mode contrast-enhanced in vivo imaging. ACS Appl Mater Interfaces, 2018, 10(38): 31947-31958.

[40] HUANG H, DU L, SU R, et al. Albumin-based co-loaded sonosensitizer and STING agonist nanodelivery system for enhanced sonodynamic and immune combination antitumor therapy. J Control Release., 2024, 375: 524-536.

[41] LIN T, ZHAO X, ZHAO S, et al. O_2-generating MnO_2 nanoparticles for enhanced photodynamic therapy of bladder cancer by ameliorating hypoxia. Theranostics, 2018, 8(4): 990-1004.

[42] WANG A, GUO M, WANG N, et al. Redox-mediated dissolution of paramagnetic nanolids to achieve a smart theranostic system. Nanoscale, 2014, 6(10): 5270-5278.

[43] ZHANG Y, TAN J, LONG M, et al. An emerging dual collaborative strategy for high-performance tumor therapy with mesoporous silica nanotubes loaded with Mn_3O_4. J Mater Chem B., 2016, 4(46): 7406-7414.

[44] ZHANG E, LUO S, TAN X, et al. Mechanistic study of IR-780 dye as a potential tumor targeting and drug delivery agent. Biomaterials, 2014, 35(2): 771-778.

[45] ZHANG E, ZHANG C, SU Y, et al. Newly developed strategies for multifunctional mitochondria-targeted agents in cancer therapy. Drug Discov Today., 2011, 16(3-4): 140-146.

[46] TONG L, CHUANG C C, WU S, et al. Reactive oxygen species in redox cancer therapy. Cancer Lett., 2015, 367(1): 18-25.

[47] MOLONEY J N, COTTER T G. ROS signalling in the biology of cancer. Semin Cell Dev Biol., 2018, 80: 50-64.

[48] YANG Z, WANG J, AI S, et al. Self-generating oxygen enhanced mitochondrion-targeted photodynamic therapy for tumor treatment with hypoxia scavenging. Theranostics, 2019, 9(23): 6809-6823.

第 3 章

近红外引导下纳米介导的线粒体呼吸抑制/损伤途径增强胃肠道恶性肿瘤的光疗效果

3.1 引言

近年来,随着临床肿瘤治疗方法和基础研究的进展,部分患者的 5 年生存率有了提高。然而不幸的是,其中大多数肿瘤患者的治疗都失败了[1-3],其中,胃肠道恶性肿瘤作为一种常见的恶性肿瘤,发病率在世界范围内位居第三位[4-5]。更糟糕的是,存在淋巴结转移的病人,5 年生存率低于 10%[6-7],这中间,对肿瘤微环境缺乏重视是治疗失败的一个重要原因。越来越多的证据表明,肿瘤不仅是宏观的肿块,其中的组织内部也涉及非常复杂的微环境成分[8-10]。肿瘤的治疗、复发、浸润和转移均与肿瘤微环境存在一定的关系[11-13],其中,以低氧浓度为突出特征的肿瘤乏氧微环境,可以通过抑制药物疗效、限制肿瘤细胞免疫浸润、促进肿瘤复发转移等手段,广泛地降低肿瘤治疗的疗效[14-18]。因此,肿瘤乏氧微环境的解除或许是减少或根治肿瘤的一种重要手段。

目前存在针对解除肿瘤乏氧微环境的各种策略,如血红蛋白和全氟化碳囊泡被用作纳米载体,直接将氧气输送至低氧环境中。然而,氧负荷低、氧漏出快、间隙压过高等因素严重制约这种方法[19-23]。此外,二氧化锰和金纳米团簇也被用于分解肿瘤组织中高表达的过氧化氢,生成氧气。但是由于可用的过氧化氢含量较低,氧气的产量还不能完全令人满意[24-27]。此外,单独的供氧方式不能持续对抗肿瘤乏氧微环境,也缺乏抑制乏氧相关信号通路的能力[28-29]。因此,寻求一个强有力解除肿瘤乏氧微环境的策略就显得尤为重要。线粒体作为细胞内重要的细胞器,在细胞内主要行使有氧呼吸的功能[30-31]。此前已有报道,肿瘤细胞的乏氧主要是由于线粒体相关氧化磷酸化过程中过量消耗氧气而导致的[32-34]。因此,对于肿瘤细胞中线粒体相关氧化磷酸化的干预也许可以抑制肿瘤细胞对氧气的消耗。

在这项研究中,我们合成了一种多功能的纳米颗粒 PEG-PCL-IR780-MET(P-P-I-M),可以通过内源性乏氧抑制和线粒体靶向的光动力疗法(Photodynamic Therapy,PDT)及光热疗法(Photothermal Therapy,PTT)实现了两阶段的抗肿瘤治疗。如图 3-1 所示,当纳米颗粒通过实体瘤的高通透性和滞留(Enhanced Permeability and Retention,EPR)效应在体内特异性地在靶向胃肠道恶性肿瘤组织后,首先抑制胃肠道恶性肿瘤细胞的线粒体呼吸(第一阶段改善肿瘤乏氧微环境),随后攻击并杀伤肿瘤细胞以及其中的线粒体,进而消灭肿瘤(第二阶段杀伤肿瘤组织)。

第3章 近红外引导下纳米介导的线粒体呼吸抑制/损伤途径增强胃肠道恶性肿瘤的光疗效果

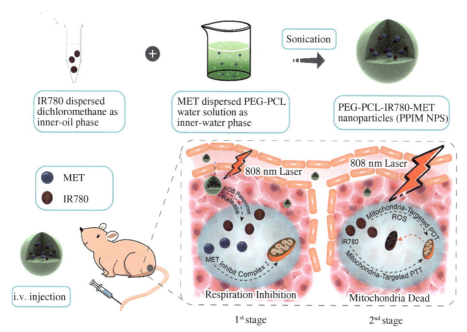

这种两阶段光疗首先抑制肿瘤组织的线粒体呼吸,随后攻击肿瘤细胞及其中的线粒体,杀伤肿瘤组织。

图 3-1 PEG-PCL-IR780-MET 纳米颗粒的设计、合成及光治疗功能的示意图

图片来自参考文献[63]

具体地说,将一种新型光敏剂 IR780(图 2-1)和二甲双胍(Metformin,MET)(图 3-2)共载于两亲性的聚乙二醇(Polyethylene Glycol,PEG)-聚己内酯(Polycaprolactone,PCL)中,合成 P-P-I-M 纳米颗粒。PEG-PCL 作为 IR780 和二甲双胍的纳米载体,具有极高的稳定性,并可通过 EPR 效应特异性地靶向肿瘤组织。基于 IR780 的光声(Photoacoustic,PA)和近红外(Near-Infrare,NIR)荧光双模态成像,证实了在静脉注射 24 h 后,肿瘤部位的纳米颗粒可达到最大的蓄积。光敏剂 IR780 使用 808 纳米激光(1 W·cm^{-2})照射肿瘤部位 1 min 后,迅速产生活性氧(Reactive Oxygen Species,ROS),并使 PEG-PCL 崩解,释放二甲双胍与 IR780。二甲双胍作为一种常用的治疗Ⅱ型糖尿病的药物,由于其极低的毒副作用而得到了美国食品药品监督管理局(Food and Drug Administration,FDA)的批准[35-36]。另据报道,二甲双胍可直接抑制线粒体电子传递链中的烟酰胺腺嘌呤二核苷酸(Nicotinamide Adenine Dinucleotide,NADH)脱氢酶的活性,从而实现对细胞呼吸的有效抑制[37-39]。从体内正电子发射计算机断层扫描（Positron Emission Computed Tomography，PET-CT）和 PA 双模态成像结果可知，在尾静脉注射 P-P-I-M 纳米颗粒 4 h 后，肿瘤的乏氧微环境受到了显著的抑制，可为肿瘤复发、转移的抑制提供有利的条件。同时，线粒体作为细胞的产生能量工厂，在肿瘤的发生、发展和转移中发挥着不可或缺的作用[40-41]。线粒体的直接破坏可能会迅速损害其生物学功能，从而加速细胞程序性死亡[42-44]。线粒体作为细胞凋亡的重要调节因素，易受 ROS 和高温诱导引起损伤[45-47]。IR780 作为一种亲脂阳离子，主要积聚在肿瘤细胞的线粒体中，在激光照射下产生 ROS 并发热，可损伤线粒体并加速胃肠道恶性肿瘤细胞的程序性死亡[48-49]。这种线粒体靶向的 PDT/PTT 协同治疗，可进一步扩大治疗效果，为胃肠道恶性肿瘤的治疗提供一种新的途径[50-53]。

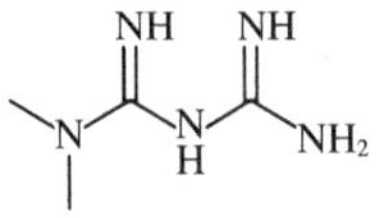

图 3-2　二甲双胍的分子结构

3.2　材料与方法

3.2.1　实验材料与仪器

1）主要实验材料

胎牛血清（Fetal Bovine Serum，FBS）、RPMI-1640 细胞培养基、无酚红 RPMI-1640 细胞培养基、胰蛋白酶、磷酸盐缓冲溶液（PBS）、链霉素、青霉素（美国 Gibco）；MitoTracker® Green FM 线粒体绿色荧光探针、LysoTracker Green DND-26 溶酶体绿色荧光探针、Calcein-AM/PI 活细胞/死细胞双染试剂盒（中国翊圣）；4%多聚甲醛固定液、活性氧检测试剂盒、细胞膜蛋白与细胞浆蛋白提取试剂盒、PVDF 膜、线粒体膜电位检测试剂盒（JC-1）、CCK-8 试剂盒（中国碧云天）；MitoCheck® Complex I Activity Assay Kit（美国 Cayman）；ROS-ID™ 乏氧/氧化应激检测试剂盒（美国 Enzo Life Sciences）；Rabbit mAb♯5174 抗 GAPDH、Rabbit mAb♯36169 抗 HIF-1α 一抗抗体（美国 Cell Signaling）；Pierce 化学发光底物（美国 Thermo Fisher）；甲氧基聚乙二醇羟基（mPEG-OH）（北京键凯）；ε-己内酯（ε-CL）、乙醚、二甲双胍、二氯甲烷（DCM）、二甲基亚砜（DMSO）、IR780（美国 Sigma-Aldrich）。

2) 主要实验仪器

二氧化碳细胞培养箱、-80 ℃实验室超低温冰箱、大容量 ST4 Plus 离心机；Ⅱ类生物安全柜（新加坡 ESCO）；玻底培养皿（中国 NEST）；纯水仪（美国 Millipore）；SX-700 高压蒸汽灭菌锅（日本 TOMY）；IX71 荧光倒置显微镜（日本 OLYMPUS）；激光共聚焦扫描显微镜（Confocal Laser Scanning Microscope，CLSM）（德国 Leica）；SpectraMax iD5-多功能酶标仪（美国 Molecular Devices）；LSRFortessa™ 流式细胞分析仪（美国 BD）；Maestro™ In-Vivo Imaging System（美国 Cri）；Nexus 128 临床前光声计算机断层扫描仪（美国 Endra）；透射电子显微镜（日本 JEOL）；动态光散射仪（英国 Malvern）；荧光分光光度计（日本 HoribaScientific）；UV-3600 紫外分光光度计（日本 Shimadzu）；ThermaCAM SC3000 红外热像仪（美国 FLIR）；Inveon Micro PET-CT system（德国 Siemens）。

3.2.2 实验方法

1) PEG-PCL 的合成

将甲氧基聚乙二醇羟基与 ε-己内酯加入真空密封体系中，在 160 ℃条件下搅拌 24 h。之后，将粗共聚物溶解到二氯甲烷中，以除去低聚物和未反应单体。最后用冷乙醚沉淀，并减压过滤干燥，得到 PEG-PCL。

2) P-P-I、P-P-M 及 P-P-I-M 纳米颗粒的合成

合成 P-P-I 纳米颗粒，首先将 50 mg PEG-PCL 溶解于 50 mL 去离子水中，超声 5 min，之后将含有 IR780（5 mg）的二氯甲烷悬浮液（10 mL）加入去离子水悬浮液中，超声 30 min。最后，用去离子水洗涤五次去除残渣，并离心获得 P-P-I 纳米颗粒。

合成 P-P-M 纳米颗粒，首先将 50 mg PEG-PCL 溶解于 50 mL 去离子水中，超声 5 min，之后将含有二甲双胍（5 mg）的 PBS 悬浮液（10 mL）加入去离子水悬浮液中，超声 30 min。最后，用去离子水洗涤五次去除残渣，并离心获得 P-P-M 纳米颗粒。

合成 P-P-I-M 纳米颗粒，首先将 50 mg 的 PEG-PCL 溶解于 50 mL 去离子水中，超声 5 min，之后将含有 IR780（5 mg）的二氯甲烷悬浮液（10 mL）和二甲双胍（5 mg）的 PBS 悬浮液（10 mL）加入去离子水悬浮液中，超声 30 min。最后，用去离子水洗涤五次去除残渣，并离心获得 P-P-I-M 纳米颗粒。

3) 形貌与表征

利用透射电子显微镜和动态光散射仪观察 P-P-I、P-P-M 及 P-P-I-M 纳米颗粒的形貌和尺寸。使用紫外分光光度计监测了这些纳米颗粒的紫外-可见吸收光谱。使用荧光分光光度计测定了 IR780、P-P-I 和 P-P-I-M 纳米颗粒的荧光光谱。每隔 12 h 监测 PBS 和血清中 P-P-I-M 纳米颗粒的粒径结果,以确定其稳定性。利用红外热像仪对这些纳米颗粒的体外光热治疗能力进行监测。在测量温度时,用锡箔包裹反应容器,以防止外部温度对其产生影响。将纳米颗粒悬浮液加入 EP 管中,用 808 nm 激光在不同条件下照射。利用 AnalyzIR 软件对温度值进行采集和分析。

4) 细胞培养

人胃癌细胞系 MKN-45P 购自中国科学院上海细胞生物学研究所。将细胞置于 RPMI-1640 培养基中,加入热灭活无菌的 FBS(10%)、青霉素(1%)和链霉素(100 g/mL),培养在 37 ℃、5% CO_2 的环境中。当细胞培养至培养皿面积约 85% 时,按照 1∶3 比例进行传代,进行之后的细胞构建与肿瘤移植瘤模型实验。

5) 胃肠道恶性肿瘤异种移植瘤模型的建立

所有动物均为 5 周龄重症联合免疫缺陷(Severe Combined Immunodeficiency,SCID)雄性 BALB/c 裸鼠,购自南京大学模式动物研究所。所有动物实验均经南京大学动物保护与利用委员会(IACUC)批准,并严格遵守《南京大学实验动物保护与利用指南》。将 MKN-45P(每只 1×10^6)细胞悬浮于 PBS(200 μL)中,皮下注射于小鼠的左上肢,建立胃肠道恶性肿瘤异种移植瘤模型。肿瘤体积按$[\pi/6\times 长\times(宽)^2]$计算。

6) 胃肠道恶性肿瘤细胞中线粒体功能的测定

使用 MitoCheck® 复合物 I 活性测定试剂盒(分为 A 管和 B 管)监测 MKN-45P 细胞内线粒体复合物 I 的活性。先将 MKN-45P 细胞与 PBS、MET 和 P-P-I-M 纳米颗粒共培养 4 h,然后加入 A 管中的混合物 50 μL。之后在每孔中加入 20 μL 分析缓冲液,并且尽可能快地加入 B 管中的混合物 30 mL。最后测量各个孔在 340 nm 处的吸光度并计算其活性。

使用 JC-1 检测试剂盒测定 MKN-45P 细胞内的线粒体膜电位。先将 MKN-45P 细胞与 PBS、MET 和 P-P-I-M 纳米颗粒共培养 4 h,之后将 JC-1 检测试剂盒加入 MKN-45P 细胞 6 孔板中,37 ℃ 培养 20 min。随后,使用 PBS 对细胞清洗三次。最后,使用流式细胞术检测正常极化的线粒体($\lambda_{ex}/\lambda_{em}=$ 525 nm/590 nm)和异常去极化线粒体($\lambda_{ex}/\lambda_{em}=$490 nm/530 nm)。

7) 胃肠道恶性肿瘤细胞中乏氧的检测

使用乏氧/氧化应激检测试剂盒检测胃肠道恶性肿瘤细胞中的乏氧情况。共分为对照、激光照射、P-P-M+激光照射、P-P-I+激光照射、P-P-I-M+激光照射 5 组。将不同纳米颗粒与 MKN-45P 细胞培养 4 h,治疗浓度以 IR780 计算,终浓度为 4 μg/mL。使用绿脓菌素(200 μM,30 分钟)作为 ROS 诱导的阳性对照,去铁胺(200 μM,4 小时)作为乏氧的阳性对照。接着按照说明书指示,将检测试剂盒中配制的混合物添加到胃肠道恶性肿瘤细胞中。共培养 30 min 后,使用 PBS 对细胞清洗三次,并在 808 nm 激光照射下对细胞进行照射。最后,使用共聚焦激光扫描显微镜(CLSM)监测 ROS 信号($\lambda_{ex}/\lambda_{em}=$488 nm/520 nm)和乏氧信号($\lambda_{ex}/\lambda_{em}=$488 nm/590 nm)。

之后,使用 Western blot 法检测 MKN-45P 细胞中缺氧诱导因子-1α(Hypoxia Inducible Factor-1α,HIF-1α)和甘油醛-3-磷酸脱氢酶(Glyceraldehyde-3-phosphate Dehydrogenase,GAPDH)的表达。使用细胞膜蛋白与细胞浆蛋白提取试剂盒提取 MKN-45P 细胞中的总蛋白,将样品转移到聚偏氟乙烯(Polyvinylidene Fluoride,PVDF)膜上。之后使用 5% 脱脂乳封闭膜,并在 8 ℃条件下与抗 GAPDH 和抗 HIF-1α 一抗孵育过夜。然后使用抗兔二抗,用 Pierce 化学发光底物使条带出现。最后采集照片,并使用 ImageJ 软件进行分析。

8) P-P-I-M 纳米颗粒的亚细胞定位

为了证明 IR780 的线粒体靶向性,分别使用荧光探针标记胃肠道恶性肿瘤细胞内的溶酶体和线粒体,以确定 P-P-I-M 的亚细胞定位。在与 P-P-I-M 纳米颗粒共培养 4 h 后,MKN-45P 细胞与溶酶体绿色荧光探针($\lambda_{ex}/\lambda_{em}=$504 nm/511 nm)共培养 30 min 标记溶酶体,或与线粒体绿色荧光探针($\lambda_{ex}/\lambda_{em}=$490 nm/516 nm)共培养 60 min 标记线粒体。之后,使用 PBS 对细胞清洗三次,并使用共聚焦激光扫描显微镜对细胞进行拍摄,获取荧光图像。利用 ImageJ 软件获得 Pearson 相关系数和共定位分析结果。

9) 胃肠道恶性肿瘤细胞内的活性氧检测

使用 H_2DC-FDA($\lambda_{ex}/\lambda_{em}=$488 nm/520 nm)活性氧检测试剂盒评估细胞内产生的活性氧。共分为对照、激光照射、P-P-I-M、P-P-M+激光照射、P-P-I+

激光照射、P-P-I-M+激光照射 6 组。将 MKN-45P 细胞接种于 6 孔板中,37 ℃ 孵育 24 h。然后将不同的纳米颗粒加入相应的孔中,治疗浓度以 IR780 计算,终浓度为 4 μg/mL。37 ℃下孵育 4 h,然后用 PBS 洗涤三次。随后,向每个孔中加入 1 mL 的活性氧检测试剂,孵育 15 min。接着将细胞洗涤三次,并用 808 nm 激光($1 W \cdot cm^{-2}$)照射 5 min,将细胞洗涤三次,用无酚红 RPMI-1640 细胞培养基重悬。最后用 CLSM 和流式细胞术观察与定量测量 ROS 的产生。

10) 体外抗肿瘤治疗效果

在证实了 P-P-I-M 具有肿瘤细胞线粒体靶向性和活性氧生成能力后,采用细胞计数法(Cell Counting Kit-8,CCK-8)和活死细胞染色法评价其体外抗肿瘤作用。实验分组和处理方式与第 9)条相同。治疗浓度以 IR780 计算,终浓度为 4 μg/mL。将癌细胞接种于培养皿(37 ℃,每孔 $1×10^4$ 个细胞)中培养 24 h,然后将不同的纳米颗粒加入相应的培养皿中,共培养 4 h。之后使用 PBS 清洗细胞三次,用 808 nm 激光($1 W \cdot cm^{-2}$)照射 5 min,再使用 PBS 清洗细胞三次。之后,按照试剂商的说明,在 MKN-45P 细胞悬液中加入 100 μL 双染色检测工作液。共培养 30 min 后,使用 PBS 清洗细胞三次。最后,用激光共聚焦显微镜观察染色后的活细胞($\lambda_{ex}/\lambda_{em}$ = 490 nm/515 nm)和死细胞($\lambda_{ex}/\lambda_{em}$ = 535 nm/617 nm)。至于 CCK-8 法,将 10 μL 试剂加入培养孔中继续共培养 4 h,按照制造商的说明,使用酶标仪在 450 nm 处测量每个孔中的吸光度值。

11) 体内近红外荧光成像

将 P-P-I-M 纳米颗粒溶解于无菌 PBS 中,通过尾静脉注射 200 μL 进入胃肠道恶性肿瘤异位移植瘤小鼠体内,浓度为 100 μg/mL。注射后 0 h、0.5 h、1 h、2 h、4 h、6 h、8 h、12 h、24 h、48 h 用 Maestro 活体荧光成像系统对这些小鼠进行成像。在 24 小时麻醉处死小鼠,获得主要器官(心、肝、脾、肺和肾)和肿瘤组织进行离体成像,进而推算纳米粒子的体内生物分布。

12) 体外和体内光声成像

使用临床前光声计算机断层扫描仪,在 700~950 nm 的波长范围内,检测波长间隔为 5 nm,使用 P-P-I-M 悬浮液进行 PA 成像,以检测纳米颗粒的最大吸光度。之后,在注射后的不同时间点(0 h、1 h、2 h、4 h、8 h、12 h、24 h 和 48 h)进行体内 PA 扫描,检测纳米颗粒的肿瘤内生物分布,P-P-I-M 的检测波长为 780 nm。

同时,注射后 24 h,光声成像监测肿瘤组织中的血管饱和氧含量,使用临床前光声计算机断层扫描仪检测肿瘤内氧合血红蛋白(850 nm)和脱氧血红蛋白(700 nm)的浓度,分析其氧合情况。

13) 活体 PET-CT 成像

为了评价不同治疗方法对胃肠道恶性肿瘤移植瘤模型的影响,将 75 μCi 的 ^{18}F-米索硝唑(^{18}F-MISO)溶解于 100 μL 的 PBS 中,并尾静脉注射于小鼠体内。之后,使用临床前 Inveon 小动物 PET-CT 系统对注射 1 小时后的小鼠进行活体正电子发射断层扫描,得到 PET 图像。所有相关数据均在工作站上进行重建和处理,计算标准摄取值(Standard Uptake Value, SUV)和相对于重量的摄取值。

14) 活体红外热成像

使用红外热像仪来检测 P-P-I-M 纳米颗粒的体内光热治疗效果。将 200 μL 的 PBS、P-P-I 纳米颗粒和 P-P-I-M 纳米颗粒尾静脉注射入胃肠道恶性肿瘤异种移植瘤模型,24 h 后,使用 808 nm 激光(1 W·cm^{-2})照射。利用红外热像仪对小鼠肿瘤部位的温度进行实时监测,并用 AnalyzIR 软件对温度值进行采集和分析。

15) 体内抗肿瘤治疗效果

将胃肠道恶性肿瘤异位移植瘤小鼠随机分为与第 9)条相同的六组,每组起始治疗时肿瘤体积约 80 mm^3。将含有不同纳米颗粒的 PBS 尾静脉注射于胃肠道恶性肿瘤异种移植瘤模型,每只 200 μL,治疗浓度以 IR780 计算,终浓度为 100 μg/mL。激光照射、P-P-M+激光照射、P-P-I+激光照射和 P-P-I-M+激光照射组的小鼠之后接受 808 nm 激光(1 W·cm^{-2})照射 5 min。然后,每两天观察小鼠情况并记录每只小鼠的体重和肿瘤体积。16 天后麻醉处死小鼠,收集肿瘤组织,用 PBS 洗涤三次,称重并用 4%多聚甲醛溶液固定。最后,用苏木精-伊红(Hematoxylin and Eosin, H-E)和 TUNEL 染色,进行免疫组织化学分析。

16) 主要器官组织病理学检测

在激光照射后,每 4 天收集小鼠的主要器官(心、肝、脾、肺和肾),用 4%多聚甲醛溶液在 4 ℃条件下固定 4 h,之后用石蜡包埋。最后,用 H-E 染色,并用光学显微镜检测组织病理学变化。

17) 血液学和血生化分析

为了评价这些纳米颗粒的生物相容性和体内毒性,每 4 天麻醉处死小鼠,采集血液进行血液学和血生化检测,包括白细胞(White Blood Cell, WBC)、中性粒细胞(Neutrophil, NEU)、淋巴细胞(Lymphocyte, LYM)、红细胞(Red

Blood Cell,RBC)、血红蛋白(Hemoglobin,HGB)、血小板(Platelet,PLT)、谷丙转氨酶(Alanine Aminotransferase,ALT)、谷草转氨酶(Aspartate Aminotransferase,AST)、血尿素氮(Blood Urea Nitrogen,BUN)和血肌酐(Serum creatinine,Scr)。

18) 统计分析

所有数据均使用 GraphPad Prism(5.01版)软件进行分析,显著性水平为:$*p<0.05$；$**p<0.01$；$***p<0.001$。所有数据均以平均值±标准差(Standard Deviation,SD)表示。

3.3 结果与讨论

3.3.1 P-P-I-M 纳米颗粒的合成与表征

根据图 3-1 的方案合成了 P-P-I-M 纳米颗粒。简单地说,一种新型光敏剂(IR780)和一种常用的糖尿病药物(MET)被包装在 PEG-PCL 脂质体中。如图 3-3(a)、(b)、(c)所示,三种不同的纳米颗粒均呈现均匀分散的球状形貌。之后,使用动态光散射仪测量了这些纳米颗粒的水合粒径。如图 3-3(d)、(e)、(f)所示,P-P-I、P-P-M 和 P-P-I-M 的平均水合粒径依次为 50.66 nm、38.83 nm 和 60.90 nm,插图为这些纳米颗粒溶解于 PBS 中的照片。如图 3-4(a)所示,MET 和 IR780 的典型吸收峰分别在 232 nm 和 789 nm 处出现。同时,在 P-P-I-M 纳米颗粒的紫外-可见-近红外光谱结果中,可以观察到 232 nm 和 789 nm 左右的两个吸收峰,表明 MET 和 IR780 已被成功加载(图 3-4(b))。此外,还检测了不同浓度下 MET 和 IR780 的紫外-可见-近红外光谱,得出标准浓度曲线(图 3-4(c)、(d))。最后,由荧光光谱结果可知,IR780 在封装入纳米颗粒后其荧光强度依然保持稳定(图 3-5)。

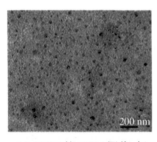

(a) P-P-I 的 TEM 图像,标尺是 200 nm

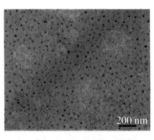

(b) P-P-M 的 TEM 图像,标尺是 200 nm

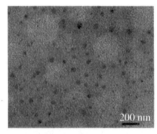

(c) P-P-I-M 的 TEM 图像,标尺是 200 nm

第 3 章　近红外引导下纳米介导的线粒体呼吸抑制/
　　　　损伤途径增强胃肠道恶性肿瘤的光疗效果

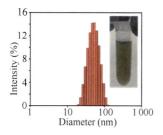 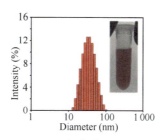 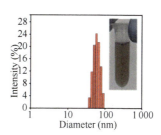

（d）P-P-I 的水合粒径,插图　　（e）P-P-M 的水合粒径,插图　　（f）P-P-I-M 的水合粒径,插图
　　为其溶解于 PBS 中的照片　　　　为其溶解于 PBS 中的照片　　　　为其溶解于 PBS 中的照片

图 3-3　不同纳米颗粒的形貌和尺寸

图片来自参考文献[63]

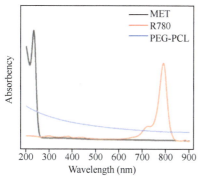 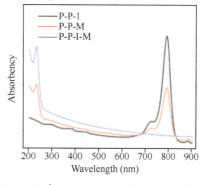

（a）二甲双胍、IR780 和 PEG-PCL　　（b）PBS 中 P-P-I、P-P-M 和 P-P-I-M 纳米
　　的紫外-可见-近红外光谱结果　　　　　颗粒的紫外-可见-近红外光谱结果

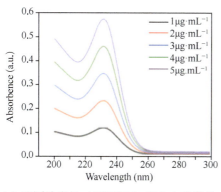 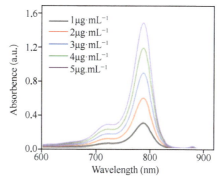

（c）不同浓度的二甲双胍在 PBS 中的紫外-　　（d）不同浓度的 IR780 在二甲基亚砜中的紫
　　可见-近红外光谱结果　　　　　　　　　　外-可见-近红外光谱结果

图 3-4　不同纳米颗粒的紫外-可见-近红外光谱结果

图片来自参考文献[63]

065

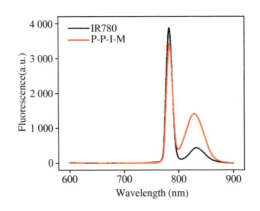

图3-5 IR780和P-P-I-M纳米颗粒的荧光光谱结果

3.3.2 P-P-I-M纳米颗粒的光疗能力测定

如图3-6(a)所示,P-P-I-M纳米颗粒的水合粒径在PBS和血清中可在约60 nm处保持稳定96 h以上,表明其具有良好的稳定性。之后,比较了在808 nm激光照射下P-P-M、P-P-I和P-P-I-M纳米颗粒的光热治疗性能。如图3-6(b)所示,P-P-I-M(从20.4 ℃到45.8 ℃)与P-P-I(从20.1 ℃到46.0 ℃)的温度上升曲线很相似。下一步确定适当的激光照射时间和功率。据文献报道,光热治疗通常需要达到50 ℃以上的高温才能取得较好的疗效[54-55]。当808 nm激光照射功率为1 W·cm^{-2}时,照射5 min后温度可以达到50.1 ℃,且1 W·cm^{-2}与1.25 W·cm^{-2}之间的温度差距不大(图3-6(c)、(d))。因此,选择使用功率为1 W·cm^{-2}的808 nm激光照射5 min作为本实验的照射方案。

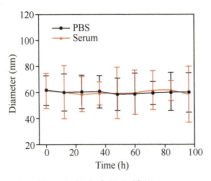

(a) 每12 h的水合粒径结果

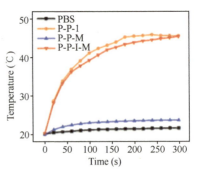

(b) 808 nm 激光照射下不同纳米颗粒的温度随时间变化的曲线

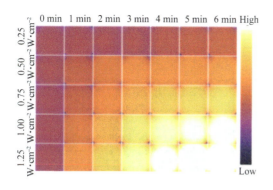
(c) 不同功率 808 nm 激光照射下 P-P-I-M 纳米颗粒的红外热像图

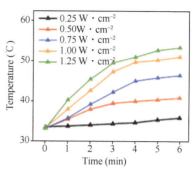
(d) 不同功率 808 nm 激光照射下 P-P-I-M 纳米颗粒的温度随时间变化的曲线

数据以平均值±标准差表示。

图 3-6 P-P-I-M 纳米颗粒的光疗能力结果

图片来自参考文献[63]

3.3.3 线粒体功能抑制及细胞毒性

首先研究 P-P-I-M 纳米颗粒是否抑制线粒体复合物Ⅰ的活性,如图 3-7(a)所示,P-P-I-M 组线粒体复合物Ⅰ的活性与 MET 组(约 60%)相似,与 PBS 组相比差异显著。然后,使用 JC-1 试剂盒进一步检测不同组中 MKN-45P 细胞线粒体膜电位的变化。如图 3-7(b)和图 3-7(c)所示,MET 和 P-P-I-M 组的细胞中存在较多的异常去极化线粒体(J-单体),而用 PBS 培养的细胞则存在更多的正常极化线粒体(J-聚集体)。之后分析 P-P-I-M 纳米颗粒的细胞毒性,如图 3-7(d)所示,三组的细胞相对存活率没有显著的统计学差异。这些结果表明,P-P-I-M 纳米颗粒能够抑制细胞线粒体复合物Ⅰ的活性,但对 MKN-45 P 细胞几乎没有细胞毒性。

3.3.4 胃肠道恶性肿瘤细胞中的乏氧情况检测

为证实 P-P-I-M 的抑制乏氧能力,使用乏氧/氧化应激检测试剂盒检测胃肠道恶性肿瘤细胞中的乏氧情况。如图 3-8 所示,绿脓杆菌组(ROS 诱导阳性对照)表现出了强烈的绿色荧光,而去铁胺组(低氧诱导剂阳性对照)表现出了较强的红色荧光,证实了这个试剂盒的有效性。由于肿瘤组织的增殖和代谢异常,许多实体瘤中存在乏氧状态[56-57]。由图 3-9(a)、(b)可知,在 PBS 组中可以检测到微弱的红色荧光,证实了肿瘤细胞的内在乏氧状态。相比较下,在 P-P-M+激光照射组基本未发现红色荧光。同时,P-P-I-M+激光照射组的 MKN-45P

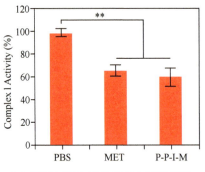
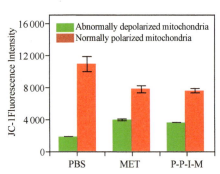

(a) PBS、MET 和 P-P-I-M 纳米颗粒与 MKN-45P 细胞共培养 4 h 后细胞线粒体复合物 I 的活性

(b) PBS、MET 和 P-P-I-M 纳米颗粒对 MKN-45P 细胞线粒体膜电位的影响

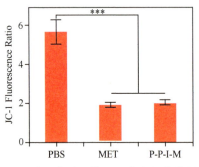
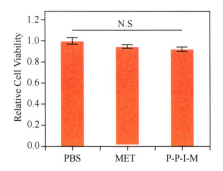

(c) 正常极化线粒体和异常去极化线粒体的比例

(d) PBS、MET 和 P-P-I-M 纳米颗粒与 MKN-45P 细胞共培养 4 h 后细胞的相对存活率

数据以平均值±标准差表示，N.S 代表没有统计学差异，** 代表 $p<0.01$；*** 代表 $p<0.001$。

图 3-7 P-P-I-M 纳米颗粒的线粒体功能抑制及细胞毒性

图片来自参考文献[63]

细胞表现最强的绿色荧光信号和最弱的红色荧光信号，而 P-P-I+激光照射组则呈现出较弱的绿色荧光和显著的红色荧光。随后的蛋白印迹结果也证实 PBS 组和激光照射组的细胞 HIF-1α 表达量中等，P-P-I+激光照射组的 HIF-1α 表达量最高。相比之下，P-P-M+激光照射组和 P-P-I-M+激光照射组由于使用 MET 而表现出了较低的 HIF-1α 水平(图 3-9(c)、(d))。基于以上结果，我们认为光敏剂如 IR780 可能通过 PDT 加重肿瘤细胞的乏氧状态，而 MET 的引入，可以抑制内源性氧的消耗，进一步克服肿瘤细胞中的乏氧，增强治疗(不仅仅是光动力治疗)的效果。

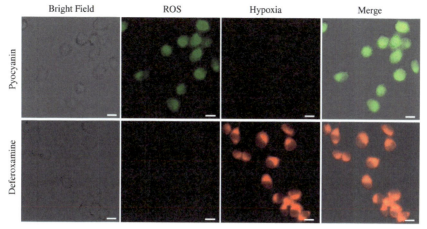

标尺是 20 μm。

图 3-8 共聚焦激光扫描显微镜检测 MKN-45P 细胞乏氧/氧化应激的状态，绿脓菌素（Pyocyanin）作为 ROS 诱导的阳性对照，去铁胺（Deferoxamine）作为乏氧的阳性对照

图片来自参考文献[63]

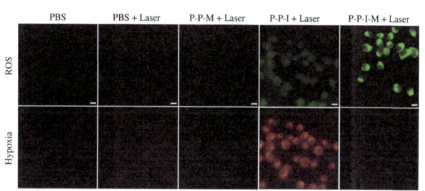

（a）使用乏氧/氧化应激检测试剂盒检测胃肠道恶性肿瘤细胞中的乏氧情况

红色荧光代表细胞乏氧，绿色荧光表示细胞中 ROS 的生成。标尺是 20 μm。

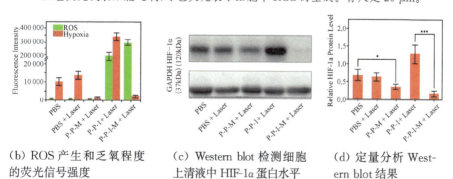

（b）ROS 产生和乏氧程度的荧光信号强度

（c）Western blot 检测细胞上清液中 HIF-1α 蛋白水平

（d）定量分析 Western blot 结果

数据以平均值±标准差表示，* 代表 $p<0.05$；*** 代表 $p<0.001$。

图 3-9 MKN-45P 细胞乏氧状态的研究

图片来自参考文献[63]

3.3.5 P-P-I-M 纳米颗粒的亚细胞定位

如前所述,IR780 作为一种亲脂阳离子,可以在肿瘤细胞内特异性结合线粒体。为了验证 IR780 从 P-P-I-M NPs 中释放后可在肿瘤细胞内特异性靶向线粒体的推测,进而发挥高效的光疗能力,我们比较了其和线粒体/溶酶体定位探针的亚细胞定位。如图 3-10(a)所示,释放后 IR780 的红色信号定位与线粒体的绿色荧光极为相似,而与溶酶体的绿色荧光不相似,其与线粒体的皮尔逊相关系数为 0.71,IR780 与溶酶体的皮尔逊相关系数为 0.25。此外,对 CLSM 结果进行共定位分析,IR780 与线粒体(图 3-10(b))表现出相似的趋势,而与溶酶体(图 3-10(c))显示出不同的趋势。因此我们得出结论,当 IR780 从纳米颗粒释放后,可以特异性地靶向线粒体,证实了线粒体靶向增强的光动力治疗是可以实现的。

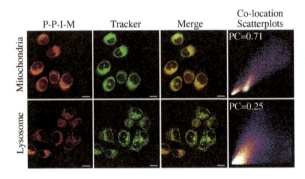

(a) 使用激光共聚焦及线粒体/溶酶体定位探针(绿色)来展示纳米颗粒的亚细胞定位,标尺是 10 μm,PC 代表皮尔逊相关系数

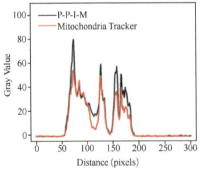

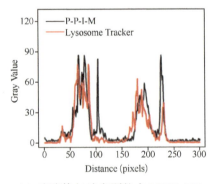

(b) 线粒体与纳米颗粒在 MKN-45P 细胞中的共定位分析

(c) 溶酶体与纳米颗粒在 MKN-45P 细胞中的共聚焦分析

图 3-10 P-P-I-M 的亚细胞定位

图片来自参考文献[63]

3.3.6 胃肠道恶性肿瘤细胞中 ROS 产量的检测

随后检测 808 nm 的激光照射下，P-P-I-M 纳米颗粒是否能在细胞内产生 ROS。将三种纳米颗粒分别与 MKN-45P 细胞共培养，之后使用 H_2DC-FDA 检测 ROS 的生成情况。如图 3-11(a)所示，经过 808 nm 激光（$1\ W \cdot cm^{-2}$）照射 5 min 后，P-P-I-M＋激光照射组的 MKN-45P 细胞内出现了强烈的绿色荧光，P-P-I＋激光组可见微弱的绿色荧光，而其余四组未见明显的绿色荧光。之后，利用流式细胞术进一步定量分析活性氧的产生情况。图 3-11(b)表现出了类似的结果，即 P-P-I-M＋激光照射组荧光强度最高，其平均荧光强度是 P-P-I＋激光照射组的 2.04 倍（图 3-11(c)），而其他组的细胞则表现出较低的绿色荧光强度。这些数据表明，随着 MET 的引入，P-P-I-M 纳米颗粒在 MKN-45P 细胞中 ROS 的产量可达到高峰，进而达到更好的 PDT 疗效。

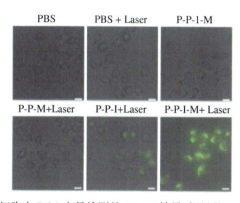

(a) 细胞中 ROS 产量检测的 CLSM 结果，标尺是 20 μm

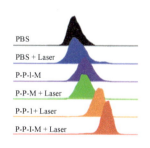

(b) 细胞中 ROS 产量检测的流式细胞术结果

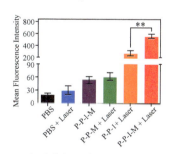

(c) 定量分析流式细胞术结果

数据以平均值±标准差表示，** 代表 $p<0.01$。

图 3-11 不同组中 MKN-45P 细胞中 ROS 产量的检测

图片来自参考文献[63]

3.3.7 体外抗肿瘤治疗效果

在证实了 P-P-I-M 纳米颗粒的 ROS 产生能力和线粒体靶向性之后,使用 Calcein-AM/PI 双染和 CCK-8 方法观察这种线粒体靶向的增强光动力治疗对于 MKN-45P 细胞的杀伤作用。如图 3-12(a)所示,P-P-M+激光照射组可观察到较多的活细胞(69.6%),表明 MET 释放后细胞毒性较小。同时,P-P-I+激光照射组的活细胞百分比约为 45.3%,与 P-P-I-M+激光照射组(16.7%)相比存在显著性差异(图 3-12(b))。之后,使用 CCK-8 法进一步检测不同组细胞的活力。如图 3-12(c)所示,PBS、激光照射和 P-P-Ⅰ-M 组中的细胞几乎完全存活。而 P-P-M+激光照射组、P-P-I+激光照射组和 P-P-I-M+激光照射组的相对细胞活力分别为 64.5%、42.9% 和 21.3%。以上结果表明,P-P-I-M 纳米颗粒在体外具有较好的生物安全性,同时可在 808 nm 激光的照射下,对于 MKN-45P 细胞具有较强的光动力治疗作用,可进一步用于体内的肿瘤治疗。

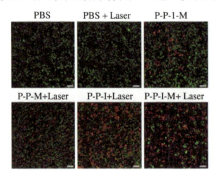

(a) 使用 Calcein-AM/PI 活死细胞双染试剂盒拍摄不同处理后细胞的 CLSM 图像。绿色荧光表示活细胞,红色荧光表示死细胞,标尺是 50 μm

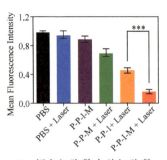

(b) 绿色细胞数占总细胞数的比例

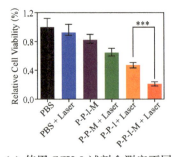

(c) 使用 CCK-8 试剂盒测定不同处理后的细胞活力

数据以平均值±标准差表示,*** 代表 $p < 0.001$。

图 3-12 不同处理后细胞毒性的检测

图片来自参考文献[63]

3.3.8 活体近红外荧光成像

体外研究后,采用胃肠道恶性肿瘤异位移植瘤模型进行体内实验。由于 IR780 具有优良的近红外荧光成像特性[58],尾静脉注射 P-P-I-M 纳米颗粒后,使用实时活体荧光成像系统在不同时间点采集实时近红外成像结果。用不同的颜色显示不同的荧光强度,荧光强度按红、黄、绿、蓝的顺序递减。如图 3-13(a)所示,注射 1 h 后可在肝脏观察到明显的荧光信号,4 h 后可在肿瘤区域观察到荧光信号,注射后 24 h 在肿瘤组织中检测到最强的荧光信号。尾静脉注射 24 h 后心、肝、脾、肺、肾和肿瘤组织的离体近红外荧光也证明了肿瘤组织具有很强烈的荧光(图 3-13(b)),肿瘤组织荧光强度较肝脏更强,且其他的主要器官中检测不到可见的荧光(图 3-13(c)),证实了这种纳米颗粒在体内对于肿瘤组织的靶向性。

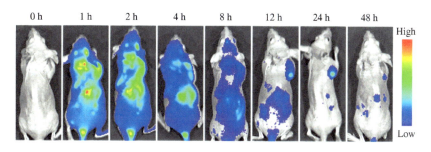

(a) 尾静脉注射 P-P-I-M 纳米颗粒后不同时间点胃肠道恶性肿瘤异位移植瘤小鼠的实时活体近红外荧光图像

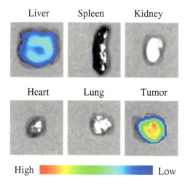

(b) 尾静脉注射 24 h 后心、肝、脾、肺、肾和肿瘤组织的离体近红外荧光

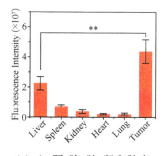

(c) 心、肝、脾、肺、肾和肿瘤组织的离体荧光信号强度

数据以平均值±标准差表示,** 代表 $p < 0.01$。

图 3-13 P-P-I-M 纳米颗粒的活体近红外荧光成像

图片来自参考文献[63]

3.3.9 光声成像结果

光声成像是近年来发展起来的一种测量组织吸收脉冲激光产生超声波的生物医学成像方法。幸运的是,IR780是一种很有前途的染料,可以用于PA成像[59-60]。如图3-14(a)所示,P-P-I-M的光声最大吸光度为780 nm。因此,可以通过光声成像在780 nm波长下进一步检测P-P-I-M纳米颗粒生物分布。如图3-14(b)和图3-14(c)所示,注射前只能观察到肿瘤局部的主要血管。随着时间的延长,肿瘤部位的光声信号逐渐增强,而肿瘤的轮廓变得更加精确。光声信号在注射后24 h达到峰值,显示出与活体近红外荧光成像相同的结果。以上结果可以证明,P-P-I-M纳米颗粒在体内可通过实体瘤的高通透性和滞留效应,特异性地在体内靶向肿瘤组织,进而降低对其他器官的非特异性毒性,并且发挥胃肠道恶性肿瘤诊断与治疗相结合的效果。

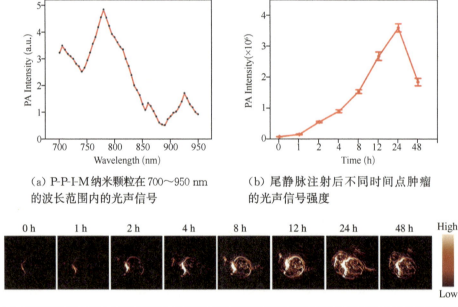

(a) P-P-I-M纳米颗粒在700~950 nm的波长范围内的光声信号

(b) 尾静脉注射后不同时间点肿瘤的光声信号强度

(c) 尾静脉注射P-P-I-M纳米颗粒后不同时间点胃肠道恶性肿瘤异位移植瘤小鼠的光声图像 数据以平均值±标准差表示。

图3-14 P-P-I-M纳米颗粒的光声成像

图片来自参考文献[63]

3.3.10 肿瘤部位PET-CT结果

为了监测P-P-I-M在体内对抗乏氧的能力,首先使用^{18}F-MISO作为PET-

CT显像剂。由于对氧的敏感性,其只能在乏氧条件下稳定地存在,因此被用作乏氧的特异标记[61-62]。由图3-15(a)可知,P-P-I+激光照射组肿瘤部位可见大量的^{18}F-MISO积累,表明肿瘤环境处于严重乏氧状态。P-P-I-M+激光照射组肿瘤区域的^{18}F-MISO信号不明显,提示肿瘤组织的乏氧情况得到了有效的缓解。之后,使用标准摄取值和相对于重量的摄取值对^{18}F-MISO信号定量。P-P-I+激光照射组(SUV:0.883±0.058;摄取:4.503% ID/g肿瘤组织)的乏氧情况比P-P-I-M+激光照射组(SUV:0.454±0.036;摄取:2.732% ID/g肿瘤组织)的乏氧情况严重很多(图3-15(b)、(c))。

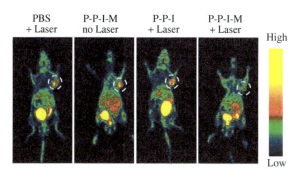

(a) 不同组的PET-CT图像

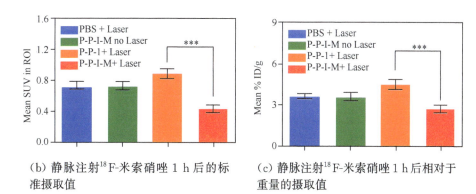

(b) 静脉注射^{18}F-米索硝唑1 h后的标准摄取值

(c) 静脉注射^{18}F-米索硝唑1 h后相对于重量的摄取值

数据以平均值±标准差表示,**代表$p<0.01$;***代表$p<0.001$。

图3-15 胃肠道恶性肿瘤异位移植瘤小鼠的PET-CT图像

图片来自参考文献[63]

3.3.11 肿瘤部位光声成像结果

进一步检测P-P-I-M纳米颗粒是否可以在体内改善肿瘤组织的乏氧状况。使用光声成像检测尾静脉注射24 h后小鼠肿瘤组织的氧合血红蛋白及脱氧血红蛋白的动态变化,实时监测肿瘤组织的含氧情况。由图 3-16(a)可知,注射后 24 h,P-P-I-M+激光照射组氧合血红蛋白含量最高,脱氧血红蛋白最低。相应地,P-P-I+激光照射组的结果正好相反。其余两组之间并没有明显差异(图 3-16(b)、(c))。这些结果表明,这种纳米颗粒可以成功地在小鼠体内增加局部氧供,进而改善肿瘤乏氧。

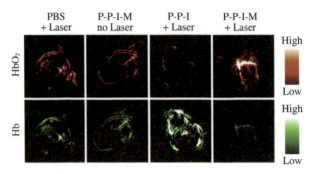

(a) 尾静脉注射 24 h 后肿瘤组织的光声成像

使用氧合血红蛋白(HbO_2)和脱氧血红蛋白(Hb)联合实时监测肿瘤组织的含氧情况。

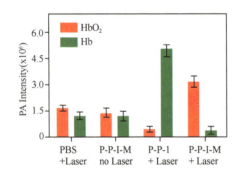

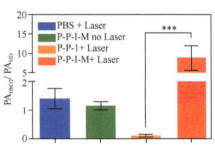

(b) 尾静脉注射 24 h 氧合血红蛋白和脱氧血红蛋白的 PA 强度

(c) 氧合血红蛋白与脱氧血红蛋白强度之比

数据以平均值±标准差表示,*** 代表 $p<0.001$。

图 3-16 胃肠道恶性肿瘤异位移植瘤小鼠不同处理后肿瘤氧合状态的检测

图片来自参考文献[63]

3.3.12 肿瘤组织 HIF-1α 免疫组化染色结果

最后,收集小鼠的肿瘤组织进行 HIF-1α 免疫组化染色,判断乏氧相关信号通路是否受到抑制(图 3-17(a))。类似地,P-P-I+激光照射组的 HIF-1α 水平

(0.853±0.112)明显高于 P-P-I-M+激光照射组(0.342±0.115),而 P-P-I-M 无激光照射组 HIF-1α 水平(0.141±0.036)与激光照射组相比无差异(0.137±0.042)(图3-17(b))。上述结果表明,常规的 PDT 或 PTT 光动力治疗可能加重肿瘤乏氧,而 MET 的引入可以抑制肿瘤乏氧微环境,进而抑制 MKN-45P 细胞的乏氧信号通路。

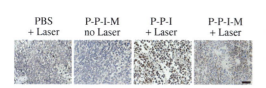

(a) 尾静脉注射 24 h 后 HIF-1α 免疫组织化学染色结果。蓝色为 HIF-1α 阴性细胞,棕色为 HIF-1α 阳性细胞,标尺是 50 μm

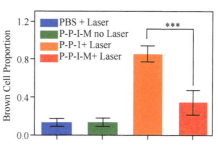

(b) HIF-1α 免疫组织化学结果中棕色细胞数占总细胞数的比例

数据以平均值±标准差表示,** 代表 $p<0.01$。

图 3-17 胃肠道恶性肿瘤异位移植瘤小鼠不同处理后的乏氧情况

图片来自参考文献[63]

3.3.13 体内抗肿瘤治疗效果

首先使用红外热成像仪检测 P-P-I-M 纳米颗粒在体内的光热治疗效果(图3-18(a))。如图3-18(b)所示,P-P-I-M+激光照射组小鼠肿瘤部位的温度从30.1 ℃迅速增加到42.8 ℃,P-P-I+激光照射组小鼠肿瘤部位的温度从28.2 ℃增加到42.4 ℃。而激光照射组小鼠肿瘤部位的温度从28.5 ℃略微升高到30.8 ℃,证实了 P-P-I-M 纳米颗粒在 808 nm 激光照射下具有较强的光热治疗效果。随后,将 MKN-45P 异位移植瘤小鼠随机分为6组,观察其对于 PDT/PTT 体内协同治疗的疗效。治疗期间各组小鼠体重无明显变化,提示这些纳米颗粒不具有明显的急性毒性(图3-18(c))。对照组肿瘤生长迅速,与第1天相比体积增加了约123倍(图3-18(d))。P-P-I+激光照射组肿瘤相对体积的增加(约4.6倍)明显低于 P-P-M+激光照射组(约7.0倍)。相比之下,P-P-I-M+激光照射组表现出强烈的抑制肿瘤体积生长(约2.4倍)的作用。第16天从小鼠体内采集到肿瘤组织的图像和重量均表现出类似的肿瘤体积变化趋势(图3-18(e)、(f))。之后,进一步用 H-E 和 TUNEL 染色研究不同治疗方法的抗肿瘤作用。H-E

切片显示,在P-P-I-M+激光照射组中,大多数肿瘤细胞被严重破坏,如核破裂、核固缩和核溶解(图3-18(g))。此外,P-P-I+激光照射组的肿瘤细胞损伤明显多于P-P-M+激光照射组。TUNEL切片中代表凋亡的暗褐色细胞核表现出了类似的结果。因此,我们推测肿瘤乏氧可能会抑制光疗的效果,导致肿瘤复发和不良预后。而P-P-I-M纳米颗粒能显著改善肿瘤乏氧微环境,进而显著抑制肿瘤的生长和复发,增强其体内PDT/PTT协同治疗的疗效。

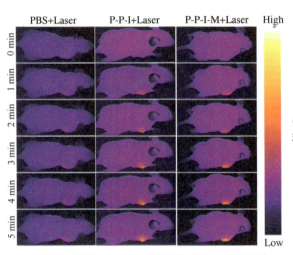

(a) 不同处理后 MKN-45P 异种移植瘤小鼠的活体红外热成像图

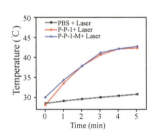

(b) 不同处理后 MKN-45P 异种移植瘤小鼠肿瘤的温度时间曲线

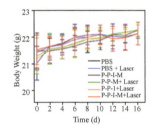

(c) 治疗 16 天的小鼠体重曲线

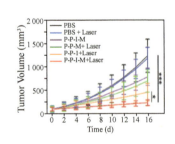

(d) 治疗 16 天的肿瘤生长曲线

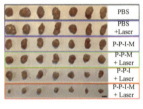

(e) 治疗 16 天后的肿瘤照片

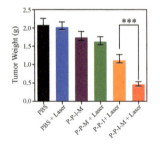

(f) 治疗 16 天后的肿瘤重量

第 3 章 近红外引导下纳米介导的线粒体呼吸抑制/损伤途径增强胃肠道恶性肿瘤的光疗效果

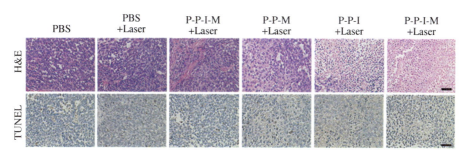

(g) 治疗 16 天后肿瘤组织的 H-E 和 TUNEL 染色结果，标尺是 50 μm

数据以平均值±标准差表示，* 代表 $p<0.05$；*** 代表 $p<0.001$。

图 3-18　不同治疗后体内抗肿瘤治疗效果检测

图片来自参考文献[63]

3.3.14　生物安全性分析

为了评估纳米颗粒的体内生物安全性，收集小鼠的心、肝、脾、肺和肾进行 H-E 染色。与对照组相比，治疗后不同时间点均表现出可忽略的炎症损伤、组织学异常以及坏死，说明 P-P-I-M 纳米颗粒具有较高的生物相容性（图 3-19(a)）。之后收集了小鼠血液进行血液学（图 3-19(b)）和血清学（图 3-19(c)）

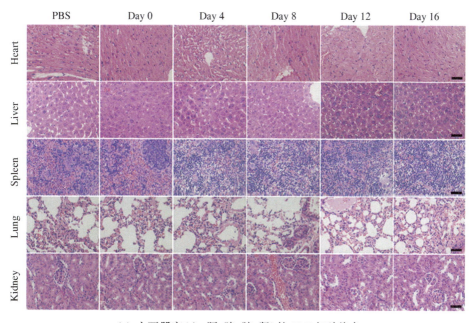

(a) 主要器官(心、肝、脾、肺、肾)的 H-E 切片染色

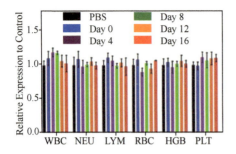 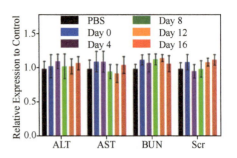

(b) 治疗期间不同时间点的血液学检查,包括白细胞(WBC)、中性粒细胞(NEU)、淋巴细胞(LYM)、红细胞(RBC)、血红蛋白(HGB)和血小板(PLT)

(c) 治疗期间不同时间点的血液学检查,包括谷丙转氨酶(ALT)、谷草转氨酶(AST)、血尿素氮(BUN)和血肌酐(Scr)。标尺是 50 μm

数据以平均值±标准差表示。

图 3-19　不同治疗后体内潜在的长期生物安全性分析

图片来自参考文献[63]

检查,以评估治疗潜在的长期生物安全性。如预期的那样,各组的免疫应答反应(WBC、NEU、LYM)、细胞毒性(RBC、HGB)、脾功能(PLT)、肝功能(ALT、AST)和肾功能(BUN、Scr)结果均未存在显著性差异。以上结果表明 P-P-I-M 纳米颗粒有很高的生物安全性,主要可能是由于肿瘤靶向给药,降低了对非肿瘤器官的副作用。

3.4　总结

本部分成功地制备了 PEG-PCL-IR780-MET(P-P-I-M)纳米颗粒以对抗肿瘤环境中的组织乏氧,进一步发挥其抗肿瘤的作用。重要的是,随着已被 FDA 批准的二甲双胍的引入,肿瘤细胞线粒体呼吸受到抑制,导致了内源性耗氧量减少。体外研究表明,P-P-I-M 能抑制线粒体复合物 I 的活性,进而抑制细胞线粒体呼吸,且细胞毒性可忽略不计。通过 ROS/乏氧双染染色、HIF-1α 水平检测、PET-CT 显像和光声成像,证实抑制细胞呼吸有助于克服肿瘤乏氧。随着 P-P-I-M 纳米颗粒在肿瘤组织中的积累,在 808 nm 激光照射下,IR780 释放并表现出优越的线粒体靶向的联合光动力和光热治疗。IR780 的特性使得通过近红外/光声双模成像实时监测生物分布并进一步指导治疗方案成为可能。此外,P-P-I-M 纳米颗粒具有良好的体内生物安全性。总之,本节证明了通过减少内源性氧消耗来对抗持续低氧限制的新方法。结合近红外/光声双模成像以及线粒体靶向增强的光动力/光热治疗,为肿瘤的诊断和治疗提供了新的思路[63]。

参考文献

[1] YANG J H, KIM H, ROH S Y, et al. Discordancy and changes in the pattern of programmed death ligand 1 expression before and after platinum-based chemotherapy in metastatic gastric cancer. Gastric Cancer, 2019, 22(1):147-154.

[2] SIEGEL R L, MILLER K D, JEMAL A. Cancer statistics, 2019. CA Cancer J Clin., 2019, 69(1):7-34.

[3] PILLERON S, SARFATI D, JANSSEN-HEIJNEN M, et al. Global cancer incidence in older adults, 2012 and 2035: a population-based study. Int J Cancer., 2019, 144(1):49-58.

[4] Torre L A, Bray F, Siegel R L, et al. Global cancer statistics, 2012. CA Cancer J Clin., 2015, 65(2):87-108.

[5] ISOBE Y, NASHIMOTO A, AKAZAWA K, et al. Gastric cancer treatment in Japan: 2008 annual report of the JGCA nationwide registry. Gastric Cancer, 2011, 14(4):301-316.

[6] KAMIYA S, TAKEUCHI H, NAKAHARA T, et al. Auxiliary diagnosis of lymph node metastasis in early gastric cancer using quantitative evaluation of sentinel node radioactivity. Gastric Cancer, 2016, 19(4):1080-1087.

[7] FERLAY J, SOERJOMATARAM I, DIKSHIT R, et al. Cancer incidence and mortality worldwide: sources, methods and major patterns in GLOBOCAN 2012. Int J Cancer., 2015, 136(5):E359-E386.

[8] GIARRATANO T, MIGLIETTA F, GIORGI CA, et al. Exceptional and durable responses to TDM-1 after trastuzumab failure for breast cancer skin metastases: potential implications of an immunological sanctuary. Front Oncol., 2018, 8:581.

[9] PIASECKA D, BRAUN M, KITOWSKA K, et al. FGFs/FGFRs-dependent signalling in regulation of steroid hormone receptors - implications for therapy of luminal breast cancer. J Exp Clin Cancer Res., 2019, 38

(1):230.

[10] REN B, CUI M, YANG G, et al. Tumor microenvironment participates in metastasis of pancreatic cancer. Mol Cancer., 2018,17(1):108.

[11] SONG M, LIU T, SHI C, et al. Bioconjugated manganese dioxide nanoparticles enhance chemotherapy response by priming tumor-associated macrophages toward M1-like phenotype and attenuating tumor hypoxia. ACS Nano., 2016,10(1):633-647.

[12] QU J, WANG Y, XIONG C, et al. In vivo gene editing of T-cells in lymph nodes for enhanced cancer immunotherapy. Nat Commun., 2024, 15(1):10218.

[13] GUO X, GUO M, CAI R, et al. mRNA compartmentalization via multi-module DNA nanostructure assembly augments the immunogenicity and efficacy of cancer mRNA vaccine. Sci Adv., 2024,10(47):3680.

[14] GAO M, LIANG C, SONG X, et al. Erythrocyte-membrane-enveloped perfluorocarbon as nanoscale artificial red blood cells to relieve tumor hypoxia and enhance cancer radiotherapy. Adv Mater., 2017, 29(35):1701429.

[15] WANG J, TIAN L, KHAN M N, et al. Ginsenoside Rg3 sensitizes hypoxic lung cancer cells to cisplatin via blocking of NF-κB mediated epithelial-mesenchymal transition and stemness. Cancer Lett., 2018,415:73-85.

[16] SALEM A, ASSELIN M C, REYMEN B, et al. Targeting hypoxia to improve non-small cell lung cancer outcome. J Natl Cancer Inst., 2018,110(1):14-30.

[17] MENG X, KONG F M, YU J. Implementation of hypoxia measurement into lung cancer therapy. Lung Cancer, 2012,75(2):146-150.

[18] HU D, CHEN L, QU Y, et al. Oxygen-generating hybrid polymeric nanoparticles with encapsulated doxorubicin and chlorin e6 for trimodal imaging-guided combined chemo-photodynamic therapy. Theranostics, 2018,8(6):1558-1574.

[19] LIU W L, LIU T, ZOU M Z, et al. Aggressive man-made red blood cells for hypoxia-resistant photodynamic therapy. Adv Mater., 2018,30(35):

e1802006.

[20] WANG S, YUAN F, CHEN K, et al. Synthesis of hemoglobin conjugated polymeric micelle: a ZnPc carrier with oxygen self-compensating ability for photodynamic therapy. Biomacromolecules, 2015, 16(9): 2693-2700.

[21] SONG X, FENG L, LIANG C, et al. Ultrasound triggered tumor oxygenation with oxygen-shuttle nanoperfluorocarbon to overcome hypoxia-associated resistance in cancer therapies. Nano Lett., 2016, 16(10): 6145-6153.

[22] CHENG Y, CHENG H, JIANG C, et al. Perfluorocarbon nanoparticles enhance reactive oxygen levels and tumour growth inhibition in photodynamic therapy. Nat Commun., 2015, 6: 8785.

[23] ZHOU Z, ZHANG B, WANG H, et al. Two-stage oxygen delivery for enhanced radiotherapy by perfluorocarbon nanoparticles. Theranostics, 2018, 8(18): 4898-4911.

[24] LEE S Y, CHOI J W, HWANG C, et al. Intravascular casting radiopaque hydrogel systems for transarterial chemo/cascade catalytic/embolization therapy of hepatocellular carcinoma. Small, 2024, 20(46): e2400287.

[25] WANG C, WANG Z, ZHAO T, et al. Optical molecular imaging for tumordetection and image-guided surgery. Biomaterials, 2018, 157: 62-75.

[26] YANG G, XU L, CHAO Y, et al. Hollow MnO_2 as a tumor-microenvironment-responsive biodegradable nano-platform for combination therapy favoring antitumor immune responses. Nat Commun., 2017, 8(1): 902.

[27] LIU C P, WU T H, LIU C Y, et al. Self-supplying O_2 through the catalase-like activity of gold nanoclusters for photodynamic therapy against hypoxic cancer cells. Small, 2017, 13(26): 10.1002/smll.201700278.

[28] YU W, LIU T, ZHANG M, et al. O_2 economizer for inhibiting cell respiration to combat the hypoxia obstacle in tumor treatments. ACS Nano., 2019, 13(2): 1784-1794.

[29] XING Y, ZHANG Y, LI J, et al. Bioresponsive nanoparticles boost starvation therapy and prevent premetastatic niche formation for pulmonary metastasis treatment. ACS Appl Mater Interfaces., 2024, 16(39): 51798-51806.

[30] XING Y, ZHANG Y, LI J, et al. Bioresponsive nanoparticles boost starvation therapy and prevent premetastatic niche formation for pulmonary metastasis treatment. ACS Appl Mater Interfaces., 2024,16(39):51798-51806.

[31] SUN C, LIU X, WANG B, et al. Endocytosis-mediated mitochondrial transplantation: transferring normal human astrocytic mitochondria into glioma cells rescues aerobic respiration and enhances radiosensitivity. Theranostics, 2019,9(12):3595-3607.

[32] MORENO-SÁNCHEZ R, RODRÍGUEZ-ENRÍQUEZ S, MARÍN-HERNÁNDEZ A. Energy metabolism in tumor cells. FEBS J., 2007, 274(6):1393-1418.

[33] MORENO-SÁNCHEZ R, MARÍN-HERNÁNDEZ A, SAAVEDRA E, et al. Who controls the ATP supply in cancer cells? Biochemistry lessons to understand cancer energy metabolism. Int J Biochem Cell Biol., 2014, 50:10-23.

[34] Grimes D R, Kelly C, Bloch K, et al. A method for estimating the oxygen consumption rate in multicellular tumour spheroids. J R Soc Interface., 2014,11(92):20131124.

[35] MORALES D R, MORRIS A D. Metformin in cancer treatment and prevention. Annu Rev Med., 2015,66:17-29.

[36] PERNICOVA I, KORBONITS M. Metformin--mode of action and clinical implications for diabetes and cancer. Nat Rev Endocrinol., 2014,10(3):143-156.

[37] Zuo H, Tao J, Shi H, et al. Platelet-mimicking nanoparticles co-loaded with $W_{18}O_{49}$ and metformin alleviate tumor hypoxia for enhanced photodynamic therapy and photothermal therapy. Acta Biomater., 2018,80:296-307.

[38] WHEATON W W, WEINBERG S E, HAMANAKA R B, et al. Metformin inhibits mitochondrial complex I of cancer cells to reduce tumorigenesis. Elife, 2014,3:e02242.

[39] Al-Qahtani Z, Al-Kuraishy H M, Ali N H, et al. Kynurenine pathway in type 2 diabetes: role of metformin. Drug Dev Res., 2024, 85

(5):e22243.

[40] Kinnally K W,Peixoto P M,Ryu S Y,et al. Is mPTP the gatekeeper for necrosis,apoptosis, or both?. Biochim Biophys Acta. , 2011,1813(4): 616-622.

[41] CHAKRABORTTY S,AGRAWALLA B K,STUMPER A,et al. Mitochondria targeted protein-puthenium photosensitizer for efficient photodynamic applications. J Am Chem Soc. , 2017,139(6):2512-2519.

[42] VANDENABEELE P,GALLUZZI L,VANDEN BERGHE T,et al. Molecular mechanisms of necroptosis: an ordered cellular explosion. Nat Rev Mol Cell Biol. , 2010,11(10):700-714.

[43] Lee D,Kim I Y,Saha S,et al. Paraptosis in the anti-cancer arsenal of natural products. Pharmacol Ther. , 2016,162:120-133.

[44] ORRENIUS S,NICOTERA P,ZHIVOTOVSKY B. Cell death mechanisms and their implications in toxicology. Toxicol Sci. , 2011,119(1):3-19.

[45] LV W,ZHANG Z,ZHANG K Y,et al. A mitochondria-targeted photosensitizer showing improved photodynamic therapy effects under hypoxia. Angew Chem Int Ed Engl. , 2016,55(34):9947-9951.

[46] YANG G, XU L, XU J, et al. Smart nanoreactors for pH-responsive tumor homing, mitochondria-targeting, and enhanced photodynamic-immunotherapy of cancer. Nano Lett. , 2018,18(4):2475-2484.

[47] WEI Y,ZHOU F,ZHANG D,et al. A graphene oxide based smart drug delivery system for tumor mitochondria-targeting photodynamic therapy. Nanoscale, 2016,8(6):3530-3538.

[48] ZHANG E,LUO S,TAN X,et al. Mechanistic study of IR-780 dye as a potential tumor targeting and drug delivery agent. Biomaterials, 2014,35(2):771-778.

[49] WANG S,GUO F,JI Y,et al. Dual-mode imaging guided multifunctional theranosomes with mitochondria targeting for photothermally controlled and enhanced photodynamic therapy in vitro and in vivo. Mol Pharm. , 2018,15(8):3318-3331.

[50] Zhao Z, Yang S, Yang P, et al. Study of oxygen-deficient $W_{18}O_{49}$-based

[51] XING R, LIU K, JIAO T, et al. An injectable self-assembling collagen-gold hybrid hydrogel for combinatorial antitumor photothermal/photodynamic therapy. Adv Mater., 2016, 28(19): 3669 - 3676.

[52] SUN N, WANG T, ZHANG S. Radionuclide-labelled nanoparticles for cancer combination therapy: a review. J Nanobiotechnology., 2024, 22(1): 728.

[53] KALLURU P, VANKAYALA R, CHIANG C S, et al. Nano-graphene oxide-mediated In vivo fluorescence imaging and bimodal photodynamic and photothermal destruction of tumors. Biomaterials, 2016, 95: 1 - 10.

[54] YOO D, JEONG H, NOH S H, et al. Magnetically triggered dual functional nanoparticles for resistance-free apoptotic hyperthermia. Angew Chem Int Ed Engl., 2013; 52(49): 13047 - 13051.

[55] JI L, HUANG J, YU L, et al. Recent advances in nanoagents delivery system-based phototherapy for osteosarcoma treatment. Int J Pharm., 2024, 665: 124633.

[56] MANKOFF D A, DUNNWALD L K, PARTRIDGE S C, et al. Blood flow-metabolism mismatch: good for the tumor, bad for the patient. Clin Cancer Res., 2009, 15(17): 5294 - 5296.

[57] EVANS J R, FENG F Y, CHINNAIYAN A M. The bright side of dark matter: lncRNAs in cancer. J Clin Invest., 2016, 126(8): 2775 - 2782.

[58] YAN J W, ZHU J Y, ZHOU K X, et al. Neutral merocyanine dyes: for in vivo NIR fluorescence imaging of amyloid-β plaques. Chem Commun., 2017, 53(71): 9910 - 9913.

[59] LI W, PENG J, YANG Q, et al. α-Lipoic acid stabilized DTX/IR780 micelles for photoacoustic/fluorescence imaging guided photothermal therapy/chemotherapy of breast cancer. Biomater Sci., 2018, 6(5): 1201 - 1216.

[60] LI X, WANG X, ZHAO C, et al. From one to all: self-assembled theranostic nanoparticles for tumor-targeted imaging and programmed photo-

active therapy. J Nanobiotechnology., 2019,17(1):23.

[61] BITTNER M I, WIEDENMANN N, BUCHER S, et al. Analysis of relation between hypoxia PET imaging and tissue-based biomarkers during head and neck radiochemotherapy. Acta Oncol., 2016,55(11):1299-1304.

[62] MAHY P, DE BAST M, DE GROOT T, et al. Comparative pharmacokinetics, biodistribution, metabolism and hypoxia-dependent uptake of [18F]-EF3 and [18F]-MISO in rodent tumor models. Radiother Oncol., 2008,89(3):353-360.

[63] YANG Z, WANG J, LIU S, et al. Defeating relapsed and refractory malignancies through a nano-enabled mitochondria-mediated respiratory inhibition and damage pathway. Biomaterials, 2020,229:119580.

第 4 章

主动靶向性氧化钨纳米颗粒介导的胃肠道恶性肿瘤双模诊断及热休克抑制的光热治疗

4.1 引言

胃肠道恶性肿瘤是世界范围内最常见的恶性肿瘤之一[1-3],每年世界范围内约有一半病例发生在东亚地区[4-5]。我国的形势更加严峻,胃肠道恶性肿瘤的发病率和死亡率均高居恶性肿瘤的第二位,且每年新发胃肠道恶性肿瘤病例绝大多为进展期[6-8]。因此,胃肠道恶性肿瘤的早期诊断以及早期的治疗干预就显得尤为重要。

光热治疗(Photothermal Therapy,PTT)作为一种新兴的无创、精确的局部治疗方法,在近年来的肿瘤治疗中得到了广泛的应用[9-10]。光热疗法能吸收近红外(Near-Infrare,NIR)光并产生热量,导致肿瘤温度升高,对肿瘤组织中的癌细胞造成不可逆转的破坏[11-12]。同时,光热疗法还具有时间空间可控制、副作用少、靶向性等优点,有望彻底替代传统的肿瘤治疗,如化疗、放疗以及手术治疗[13-15]。目前已有的一些纳米颗粒被合成为光热治疗肿瘤的药物,如硫化铜(CuS)纳米颗粒、有机纳米颗粒、石墨烯和金纳米颗粒等[16-20]。尽管如此,PTT的治疗效果仍受到多种因素的影响,包括肿瘤部位蓄积量不足、光热转换效率不高及肿瘤细胞耐热性强,从而不能完全杀死癌细胞并导致肿瘤的复发[21-23]。此外,由于缺乏有效的实时技术来监测治疗效果,使得光热治疗在临床上进一步的推广变得困难。因此,迫切地需要开发一种有效的方法来增强光热治疗的抗肿瘤作用并且可实时监测其治疗效果。

目前,由于肿瘤组织的渗透性和聚集性较差,许多抗肿瘤方法在临床上难以进一步推广。而靶向抗体和多肽,包括血管内皮生长因子(Vascular endothelial growth factor,VEGF)、人表皮生长因子受体-2(Human Epidermal Growth Factor receptor-2,HER-2)和精氨酸-甘氨酸-天冬氨酸(Arg-Gly-Asp,RGD)肽,由于具有高度的生物相容性和对肿瘤的特异性,可能有助于解决这一问题[24-29]。然而,传统的靶向肽只是将药物输送到肿瘤区域的血管,而没有帮助渗透到肿瘤组织以及细胞中。不幸的是,许多抗肿瘤药物在肿瘤细胞中的渗透量很低,只有3~5个细胞直径,从而导致实体瘤的耐药性较强进而导致较差的疗效[30-31]。最近发现的一种具有肿瘤靶向性的带有N端半胱氨酸的环型多肽iRGD (CRGDK/RGPD/EC)(图4-1)可以同时解决这些问题[32-33]。首先,iRGD可与肿瘤新生血管内皮细胞中特异性高表达的整合素 $\alpha_v\beta_3$ 受体结合,进而

第4章 主动靶向性氧化钨纳米颗粒介导的胃肠道恶性肿瘤双模诊断及热休克抑制的光热治疗

特异性地靶向肿瘤组织。之后,iRGD 被肿瘤相关蛋白酶进行分解,进而基于其 C 端的序列(R/KXXR/K)暴露,使得其获得了针对神经肽-1(Neuropilin-1, NRP-1)的亲和力。之后,其 C 端的序列进一步与 NRP-1 结合,从而触发细胞内化并导致组织渗透[34-35]。因此,结合 iRGD 可显著增强纳米颗粒的靶向性,提高抗肿瘤药物的治疗效果。

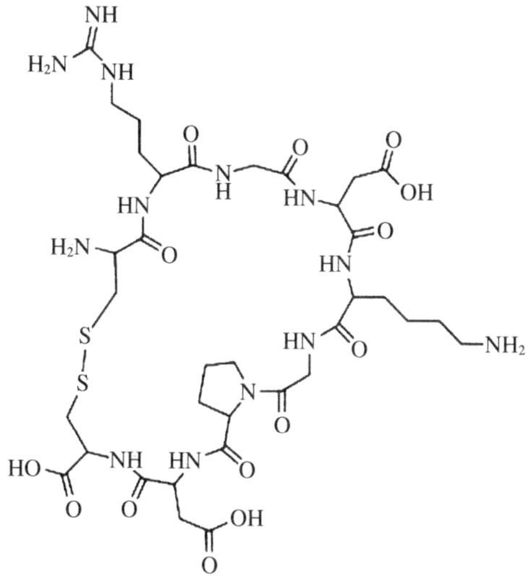

图 4-1 iRGD 的分子结构

肿瘤细胞能激活细胞保护和抗凋亡途径,如热休克反应,从而产生热阻抗并抵御光热治疗的效果,进而达到存活的作用。热休克反应可直接导致热休克蛋白(Heat Shock Proteins, HSPs)包括 HSP110、HSP90 和 HSP70 的应激性过度表达[36-38]。由于热休克蛋白对肿瘤的存活和生长有明显的促进作用,一些热休克蛋白抑制剂被开发出来以拮抗热休克蛋白的作用,进而提高肿瘤治疗的疗效[39-40]。坦螺旋霉素(Tanespimycin, 17-Allylamino-17-demethoxygeldanamycin)即 17AAG(图 4-2),是一种 HSP90 抑制剂,可以特异性地与 HSP90 的 ATP 囊相结合,从而破坏其热保护功能,进而导致癌细胞死亡[41-42]。因此,将 17AAG 与光热治疗相结合,可以克服肿瘤对于 PTT 的耐热性,进而提高 PTT 的疗效,具有广阔的应用前景。

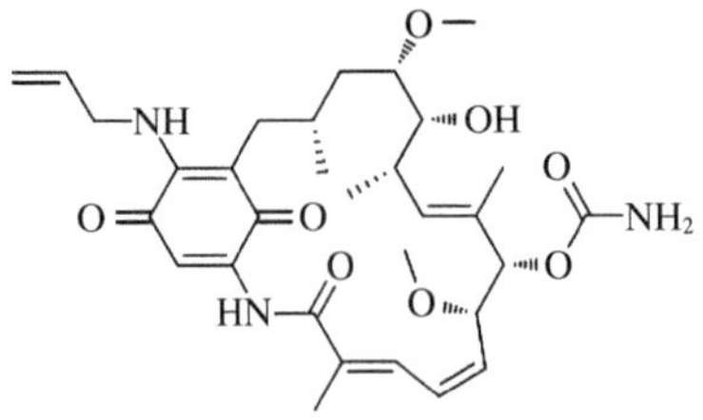

图 4-2　17AAG 的分子结构

此外,影像引导下的癌症治疗越来越引起人们的关注,因为它可以揭示肿瘤的位置、大小、实时评估治疗反应和最佳治疗时间窗等关键细节[43]。因此,影像学引导下的治疗在诊断肿瘤发生、指导光疗和监测治疗效果方面显示出巨大的潜力。作为一种有效的诊断工具,计算机断层扫描(Computed Tomography,CT)由于其具有优秀的扫描密度($\geqslant 50~\mu m$)及空间分辨率,能够提供很多的临床特征信息,并能对解剖细节进行三维成像重建[44-46]。然而,CT 成像也受制于软组织敏感性差和实时成像能力不足等限制。近红外荧光成像是一种新兴的生物医学成像方法,由于其无创性和高灵敏度等优点,可以一定程度上弥补 CT 的缺点[47-49]。此外,近红外荧光成像可以实时监测成像剂的体内生物分布。因此相较于分别的单独应用,将 CT 与近红外荧光成像相结合具有互补优势,有利于治疗的监测和指导。

基于以上设计,如图 4-3 所示,设计合成了包含羧基功能化的 $W_{18}O_{49}$ 纳米粒子、整合素靶向肽 iRGD 和 HSP90 抑制剂 17AAG 的具有胃肠道恶性肿瘤主动靶向性的多功能诊疗一体化纳米粒子(iRGD-$W_{18}O_{49}$-17AAG)。根据以往的研究,$W_{18}O_{49}$ 纳米颗粒具有较高的光热转换性能、较低的无机纳米材料代谢率和体内外生物安全性,可作为理想的 PTT 载体[50-52]。此外,作为一种金属纳米粒子,$W_{18}O_{49}$ 纳米颗粒具有很强的吸收 X 射线的能力,可以作为 CT 成像造影剂[53-54]。新型的带有 N 端半胱氨酸的环型多肽相较于传统 RGD 多肽,保留了其整合素靶向性,且具有更高的肿瘤细胞穿透效率。同时,17AAG 可以通过酯化作用与 $W_{18}O_{49}$ 纳米颗粒相结合,从而抑制胃肠道恶性肿瘤细胞的热休克反应,克服其耐热性,进而通过光热治疗的作用来提高抗肿瘤的效率。且纳米粒子 iRGD-$W_{18}O_{49}$-17AAG 经过菁 5.5 胺(Cyanine 5.5 Amine,Cy5.5)染料(图 4-4)修饰后,具有了近红外荧光成像的功能,可使用 CT/NIR 荧光双模成像来诊断肿瘤并监测纳米颗粒的体内外生物分布。细胞内近红外荧光检测、活体近红外荧光成像和活体 CT 成像证实 iRGD-$W_{18}O_{49}$-17AAG 纳米颗粒在体内及体外具有较强的肿瘤靶向性。之后的体外和体内抗肿瘤实验也表明了其在 17AAG 的帮助下可更有效地杀伤肿瘤组织。这是首次以 $W_{18}O_{49}$ 纳米颗粒为核心,通过抑制热休克反应来克服肿瘤组织的耐热性,进而增强 808 nm 激光照射下光热治疗的效果。总之,在 CT/NIR 荧光双模成像的指导下,iRGD-$W_{18}O_{49}$-17AAG 可以在肿瘤组织中聚集,进而穿透癌细胞,抑制热休克反应,从而增强光热治疗的效果,实现对恶性肿瘤组织的精准消融。

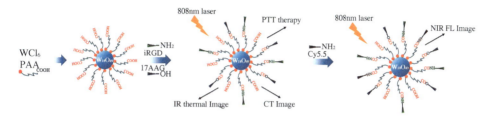

图 4-3　iRGD-$W_{18}O_{49}$-17AAG 的合成方法示意图

图片来自参考文献[60]

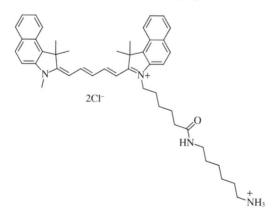

图 4-4　菁 5.5 胺(Cy5.5)染料的分子结构

4.2　材料与方法

4.2.1　实验材料与仪器

1) 主要实验材料

胎牛血清(Fetal Bovine Serum,FBS)、RPMI-1640 细胞培养基、无酚红 RP-

MI-1640细胞培养基、胰蛋白酶、磷酸盐缓冲溶液(Phosphate Buffered Saline, PBS)、链霉素、青霉素(美国 Gibco); Calcein-AM/PI 活细胞/死细胞双染试剂盒(中国翊圣); 4%多聚甲醛固定液、CCK-8试剂盒(中国碧云天); iRGD(CRGD-KGPDC)(中国 Bankpeptide); 17AAG(美国 Alexis); Cyanine 5.5 Amine (Cy5.5)(中国凯新生物); 六氯化钨(Tungsten Hexachloride, WCl_6)、聚丙烯酸(Poly Acrylic Acid, PAA)、二甘醇(Diethylene Glycol, DEG)、二甲基亚砜(DMSO)、乙基二甲氨基丙基碳化二亚胺(Ethyl Dimethylaminopropyl Carbodiimide, EDC)和 N-羟基硫代琥珀酰亚胺(Sulfo-NHS)(美国 Sigma-Aldrich)。

2) 主要实验仪器

二氧化碳细胞培养箱、−80 ℃实验室超低温冰箱、大容量ST4 Plus离心机、ESCALAB-250 X射线光电子能谱仪(美国 Thermo Fisher); Ⅱ类生物安全柜(新加坡 ESCO); 玻底培养皿(中国 NEST); 纯水仪(美国 Millipore); SX-700高压蒸汽灭菌锅(日本 TOMY); IX71荧光倒置显微镜(日本 OLYMPUS); 激光共聚焦扫描显微镜(Confocal Laser Scanning Microscope, CLSM)(德国 Leica); SpectraMax iD5-多功能酶标仪(美国 Molecular Devices); LSRFortessa™流式细胞分析仪(美国 BD); Maestro™ In-Vivo Imaging System(美国 Cri); 透射电子显微镜、高分辨率透射电子显微镜(日本 JEOL); 动态光散射仪(英国 Malvern); NexION 300D ICP - MS(美国 PerkinElmer); 粉末X射线衍射仪(日本 Rigaku); UV-3600紫外分光光度计(日本 Shimadzu); ThermaCAM SC3000红外热像仪(美国 FLIR); B13-3智能恒温数显磁力搅拌器(杭州佑宁); Clinical Gemstone spectral 64-Detector CT(美国 GE Amersham); Hiscan XM Micro CT System(中国海斯菲德)。

4.2.2 实验方法

1) 羧基功能化 $W_{18}O_{49}$ 纳米粒子的合成

首先以DEG为溶剂,制备羧基功能化 $W_{18}O_{49}$ 纳米粒子。简单来说,将 WCl_6(600 mg)与PAA(200 mg)溶解于DEG(50 mL)中,将悬浮液升温至160 ℃保持30 min,然后冷却至25 ℃。之后,将混合物加入去离子水(50 mL)中,以诱导沉淀。最后,离心混合物,用去离子水洗涤沉淀三次以除去残渣,并冻干收集羧基功能化的 $W_{18}O_{49}$ 纳米粒子。

2) iRGD-$W_{18}O_{49}$-17AAG纳米颗粒及其中间产物的合成

根据设计,iRGD和17AAG均是通过连接 $W_{18}O_{49}$ 纳米粒子上活化的羧基达到合成的效果。简单来说,在含有 $W_{18}O_{49}$ 纳米粒子(80 mg)的去离子水(50 mL)中,加入 EDC(100 mg)和 Sulfo-NHS(75 mg),随后在上述悬浮液中加入浓度为 1 mg/mL 的 iRGD 或 17AAG 或 iRGD/17AAG 的 DMSO(50 mL)。之后,使用磁力搅拌器在 4 ℃情况下搅拌 12 h。最后,离心混合物,用去离子水洗涤沉淀三次以除去多余的 iRGD 和 17AAG,并冻干得到 iRGD-$W_{18}O_{49}$、$W_{18}O_{49}$-17AAG 和 iRGD-$W_{18}O_{49}$-17AAG 纳米颗粒。

3) Cy5.5 修饰的 iRGD-$W_{18}O_{49}$-17AAG 纳米颗粒的合成

修饰 iRGD-$W_{18}O_{49}$-17AAG 纳米颗粒的方法与第 2)条类似,简单来说,在含有 $W_{18}O_{49}$ 纳米粒子(16 mg)的去离子水(10 mL)中,加入 EDC(20 mg)和 Sulfo-NHS(15 mg),随后在上述悬浮液中加入浓度为 1 mg/mL Cy5.5 的 DMSO(50 mL)。之后,使用磁力搅拌器在 4 ℃情况下搅拌 12 h。最后,离心混合物,用去离子水洗涤沉淀三次以除去多余残渣,并冻干得到 Cy5.5 修饰的 iRGD-$W_{18}O_{49}$-17AAG 纳米颗粒。

4) 形貌与表征

使用透射电子显微镜(Transmission Electron Microscopy, TEM)、高分辨透射电子显微镜和动态光散射(Dynamic Light Scattering, DLS)研究了 $W_{18}O_{49}$、iRGD-$W_{18}O_{49}$、$W_{18}O_{49}$-17AAG 和 iRGD-$W_{18}O_{49}$-17AAG 纳米材料的形貌与尺寸。每隔 10 h,测定 iRGD-$W_{18}O_{49}$-17AAG 纳米颗粒在 PBS 和血清中 DLS 结果,观察其稳定性,所有试验一式三份。使用 X 射线光电子能谱(X-ray Photoelectron Spectroscopy, XPS)结果测定了 $W_{18}O_{49}$ 纳米颗粒冻干粉末表面的元素组成。采用 X 射线衍射(X-ray Diffraction, XRD)技术测定其在 10°到 60°的 2θ 范围。利用傅里叶变换红外光谱(Fourier Transform Infrared, FTIR)研究了上述纳米颗粒冻干后的透射比变化。使用紫外-可见-近红外(Ultraviolet-visible-Near-Infrared, UV-vis-NIR)光谱结果测定了 $W_{18}O_{49}$ 纳米颗粒和 17AAG 在去离子水及 DMSO 中的浓度。17AAG 的标准浓度曲线是使用 UV-vis-NIR 结果中 320 nm 波长下的吸收值绘制的。

5) 细胞培养

从中国科学院上海细胞生物学研究所获取 MKN-45P 细胞(人胃癌细胞系)和 GES-1 细胞(人胃上皮细胞系),RPMI-1640 细胞培养基中添加了无菌的 FBS(10%)、青霉素(1%)和链霉素(100 g/mL),培养在 37 ℃、5% CO_2 的环境中。当细胞培养至培养皿面积约85%时,按照1∶3比例进行传代。

6) 胃肠道恶性肿瘤异位移植瘤模型的建立

从南京大学模式动物研究所购得4周龄重症联合免疫缺陷(Severe Combined Immunodeficiency, SCID)雄性BALB/c裸鼠。所有动物实验均经南京大学动物保护与利用委员会(IACUC)批准,并严格遵守《南京大学实验动物保护与利用指南》。为建立胃肠道恶性肿瘤异位移植瘤模型,将MKN-45P(1×10^7每只)细胞悬浮于PBS(200 μL)中,皮下注射于裸鼠左腿侧,肿瘤体积按[$\pi/6\times$长$\times$(宽)^2]计算。

7) 胃肠道恶性肿瘤细胞的选择性摄取

使用流式细胞仪检测对于iRGD-$W_{18}O_{49}$-17AAG纳米颗粒的选择性摄取的能力。将MKN-45P和GES-1细胞以每孔1×10^6的密度接种到六孔板中,培养24 h后,用PBS洗涤细胞三次。之后用1 mL经Cy5.5($\lambda_{ex}/\lambda_{em}$=684 nm/710 nm)修饰的iRGD-$W_{18}O_{49}$-17AAG纳米颗粒与细胞共培养4 h,然后使用PBS洗涤MKN-45P和GES-1细胞各三次,随后使用胰蛋白酶消化处理。最后,将细胞分离并悬浮于PBS中,使用流式细胞仪获得实验结果。

8) 体内生物分布与近红外荧光成像

将iRGD-$W_{18}O_{49}$-17AAG纳米颗粒溶解于无菌PBS中,通过尾静脉注射入胃肠道恶性肿瘤异位移植瘤小鼠体内,浓度为每只小鼠100 μL(钨1 mg/mL)。注射后0 h、1 h、4 h、12 h、24 h、48 h用Maestro活体荧光成像系统对这些小鼠进行成像。在24 h麻醉处死小鼠,获得主要器官(心、肝、脾、肺和肾)和肿瘤组织进行离体成像。同时,在尾静脉注射1 h、4 h、12 h、24 h、48 h后麻醉处死小鼠。收集肿瘤组织和主要器官,称重并在王水中溶解。使用电感耦合等离子体质谱(Inductively Coupled Plasma Mass Spectrometry, ICP-MS)测定其中锰的含量,进而推算纳米粒子的体内生物分布。

9) 体内外CT成像

首先,将临床上常用的碘造影剂碘丙醇(碘浓度分别为3.125 mM、6.25 mM、12.5 mM、25 mM、50 mM、100 mM)悬浮液和iRGD-$W_{18}O_{49}$-17AAG纳米颗粒(钨浓度分别为3.125 mM、6.25 mM、12.5 mM、25 mM、50 mM、100 mM)悬浮液加入EP管中。之后使用临床64排螺旋CT采集碘丙醇和iRGD-$W_{18}O_{49}$-17AAG纳米颗粒的体外CT图像,X射线管设置为电流400 μA,电压为70 kV。

之后小鼠尾静脉注射 iRGD-$W_{18}O_{49}$-17AAG 纳米颗粒悬浮液,浓度为每只小鼠 100 μL(钨 1 mg/mL)。注射后 24 h 使用海斯菲德微型 CT 扫描小鼠,X 射线管设置为电流 133 μA,电压为 60 kV。最后,使用海斯菲德重建软件重建图像,并用海斯菲德分析软件对图像结果进行分析。

10) 体内外红外热成像

使用 ThermaCAM 红外热像仪分析 iRGD-$W_{18}O_{49}$-17AAG 纳米颗粒的体外光热治疗能力。将 iRGD-$W_{18}O_{49}$-17AAG(钨 1 mg/mL)悬浮液加入 EP 管中,在 808 nm 激光照射下,每 50 s 采集一次红外热像图。之后采集小鼠的体内红外热成像图。小鼠尾静脉注射 100 μL PBS、$W_{18}O_{49}$-17AAG 纳米颗粒及 iRGD-$W_{18}O_{49}$-17AAG 纳米颗粒悬浮液,浓度为每只小鼠钨浓度 1 mg/mL。在注射 24 h 后,使用 808 nm 激光(2 W·cm^{-2})照射 5 min,利用红外热像仪对实时的温度变化进行检测。利用 AnalyzIR 软件对温度值进行采集和分析。

11) 体外抗肿瘤治疗效果

采用细胞计数法(Cell Counting Kit-8,CCK-8)和活死细胞染色法评价其体外抗肿瘤作用。将 MKN-45P 细胞接种于 96 孔板中 12 h。共分为对照、激光照射、iRGD-$W_{18}O_{49}$-17AAG、$W_{18}O_{49}$-17AAG+激光照射、iRGD-$W_{18}O_{49}$+激光照射和 iRGD-$W_{18}O_{49}$-17AAG+激光照射 6 组。治疗浓度以钨浓度计算,终浓度为 1 mg/mL。37 ℃下孵育 4 h,之后用 PBS 洗涤三次。用 808 nm 激光(2 W·cm^{-2})照射 5 min,将细胞洗涤三次。之后,按照试剂商的说明,在 MKN-45P 细胞悬液中加入 100 μL 双染色检测工作液。共培养 30 min 后,使用 PBS 清洗细胞三次。最后,用激光共焦显微镜观察染色后的活细胞($\lambda_{ex}/\lambda_{em}$=490 nm/515 nm)和死细胞($\lambda_{ex}/\lambda_{em}$=535 nm/617 nm)。至于 CCK-8 法,将 10 μL 试剂加入培养孔中继续共培养 4 h,按照制造商的说明,使用酶标仪在 450 nm 处测量每个孔中的吸光度值。根据说明书指示计算不同处理下的细胞数量。

12) 体内抗肿瘤治疗效果

为评价 iRGD-$W_{18}O_{49}$-17AAG 的体内抗肿瘤作用,建立胃肠道恶性肿瘤异位移植瘤模型。当肿瘤体积达到约 100 mm^3 时,将胃肠道恶性肿瘤异位移植瘤小鼠随机分为与第 11)条相同的六组,每组 5 只鼠。将含有不同纳米颗粒的 PBS 尾静脉注射于胃肠道恶性肿瘤异种移植瘤模型中,治疗浓度以钨元素计算,浓度为每只小鼠 100 μL(钨 1 mg/mL)。激光照射、$W_{18}O_{49}$-17AAG+激光照射、iRGD-$W_{18}O_{49}$＋激光照射和 iRGD-$W_{18}O_{49}$-17AAG＋激光照射组的小鼠之后接受 808 nm 激光(2 W·cm^{-2})照射 5 min。然后,每两天观察小鼠情况并记录每只小鼠的体重和肿瘤体积。16 天后麻醉处死小鼠,收集肿瘤组织,用 PBS 洗涤三次,拍照、称重并用 4%多聚甲醛溶液固定。最后,用苏木精-伊红(Hematoxylin and Eosin,H-E)和 TUNEL 染色,进行免疫组织化学分析。

13) 生物安全性分析

在治疗 16 天后麻醉处死小鼠,收集主要器官(心、肝、脾、肺和肾),用 4%多聚甲醛溶液在 4 ℃条件下固定 4 h,之后用石蜡包埋。最后,用 H-E 染色,并用光学显微镜检测组织病理学变化。随后,血液学和血生化分析也被用来评价 iRGD-$W_{18}O_{49}$-17AAG 的体内毒性以及生物相容性。治疗后第 16 天,麻醉处死小鼠,采集小鼠血液进行血液学和血生化检测,包括白细胞(White Blood Cell,WBC)、中性粒细胞(Neutrophil,NEU)、淋巴细胞(Lymphocyte,LYM)、红细胞(Red Blood Cell,RBC)、血红蛋白(Hemoglobin,HGB)、血小板(Platelet,PLT)、谷丙转氨酶(Alanine Aminotransferase,ALT)、谷草转氨酶(Aspartate Aminotransferase,AST)、血尿素氮(Blood Urea Nitrogen,BUN)和血肌酐(Serum creatinine,Scr)。

14) 统计分析

所有数据均使用 GraphPad Prism(5.01 版)软件进行分析,显著性水平为: $*p<0.05$;$**p<0.01$;$***p<0.001$。所有数据均以平均值±标准差(Standard Deviation,SD)表示。

4.3 结果与讨论

4.3.1 iRGD-$W_{18}O_{49}$-17AAG 的合成与表征

首先证明 $W_{18}O_{49}$ 纳米颗粒的合成成功。如图 4-5(a)所示,$W_{18}O_{49}$ 纳米颗粒的高分辨率透射电镜图可见其晶格间距为 0.38 nm,可以对应其(010)晶格。X 射线衍射结果表明,所合成纳米颗粒内所有的峰均对应于粉末衍射标准联合委员会(Joint Committee on Powder Diffraction Standards,JSPDC)编号 712450 对应的单斜相,也可进一步证明所合成的物质为 $W_{18}O_{49}$ 纳米颗粒(图 4-5(b))。之后,使用 X 射线光电子能谱分析 $W_{18}O_{49}$ 纳米颗粒冻干粉末的表面的元素组成。如图 4-5(c)所示,结果中可检测到钨(W)、碳(C)和氧(O)三种元素的峰,也可证实

第4章 主动靶向性氧化钨纳米颗粒介导的胃肠道恶性肿瘤双模诊断及热休克抑制的光热治疗

$W_{18}O_{49}$ 纳米颗粒的成功合成。最后,使用分光光度法测定了 $W_{18}O_{49}$ 纳米颗粒的紫外-可见-近红外光的吸光度。如图 4-5(d)所示,$W_{18}O_{49}$ 纳米颗粒的吸收强度随着波长的增加而逐渐增大,证实了其可以用作光热治疗的核心。

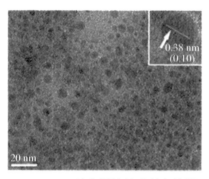

(a) $W_{18}O_{49}$ 纳米颗粒的透射电镜图片。插图为高分辨率透射电镜图片,晶格间距为 0.38 nm

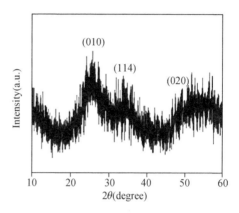

(b) $W_{18}O_{49}$ 纳米颗粒的 XRD 结果

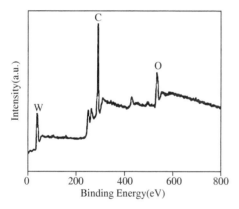

(c) $W_{18}O_{49}$ 纳米颗粒的 XPS 结果

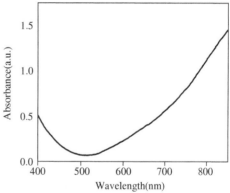

(d) $W_{18}O_{49}$ 纳米颗粒的紫外-可见-近红外光谱结果

图 4-5 $W_{18}O_{49}$ 纳米颗粒的表征

图片来自参考文献[60]

之后测定 iRGD-$W_{18}O_{49}$-17AAG 及其相关纳米颗粒的形貌和尺寸。如图 4-6(a)、(b)、(c)和(d)所示,所有纳米粒子均呈均匀分散的球形,平均粒径依次约为 10 nm($W_{18}O_{49}$)、65 nm(iRGD-$W_{18}O_{49}$)、35 nm($W_{18}O_{49}$-17AAG)和 120 nm(iRGD-$W_{18}O_{49}$-17AAG)。随后使用动态光散射仪测量纳米粒子的水合

粒径。如图 4-6(e)和(f)所示,纳米颗粒的平均水合粒径依次约为 12 nm($W_{18}O_{49}$)、78 nm(iRGD-$W_{18}O_{49}$)、40 nm($W_{18}O_{49}$-17AAG)和 135 nm(iRGD-$W_{18}O_{49}$-17AAG)。实际上,纳米颗粒的尺寸在纳米药物的设计中起着至关重要的作用。一般小于 10 nm 的颗粒通常通过肾脏代谢,而大于 200 nm 的颗粒则可以通过肝脏或脾脏过滤出体内,因此据文献报道,纳米药物的粒径在 10 nm 至 200 nm 之间是可避免肾脏清除的理想尺寸,从而可以提供合适的生物分布以及有效地在肿瘤组织中的蓄积[55-57]。

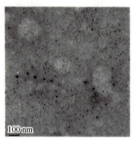
(a) $W_{18}O_{49}$ 纳米颗粒的 TEM 图像,标尺是 100 nm

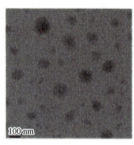
(b) iRGD-$W_{18}O_{49}$-17AAG 纳米颗粒的 TEM 图像,标尺是 100 nm

(c) iRGD-$W_{18}O_{49}$ 纳米颗粒的 TEM 图像,标尺是 100 nm

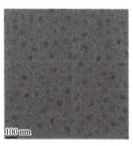
(d) $W_{18}O_{49}$-17AAG 纳米颗粒的 TEM 图像,标尺是 100 nm

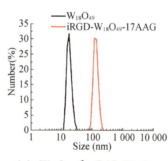
(e) $W_{18}O_{49}$ 和 iRGD-$W_{18}O_{49}$-17AAG 纳米颗粒水合粒径

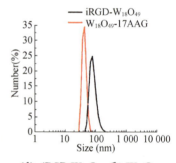
(f) iRGD-$W_{18}O_{49}$ 和 $W_{18}O_{49}$-17AAG 纳米颗粒的水合粒径

图 4-6 不同纳米颗粒的形貌和尺寸

图片来自参考文献[60]

之后,使用傅里叶变换红外光谱结果证实了 iRGD-$W_{18}O_{49}$-17AAG 纳米颗粒的成功合成。如图 4-7(a)所示,$W_{18}O_{49}$ 纳米颗粒在 3 350 cm^{-1} 处可见典型的羧基吸收峰。而 iRGD-$W_{18}O_{49}$-17AAG 纳米颗粒的傅里叶变换红外光谱结果中,羧基吸收峰明显降低,说明 $W_{18}O_{49}$ 表面的活性羧基被 iRGD 和 17AAG

第4章 主动靶向性氧化钨纳米颗粒介导的胃肠道恶性肿瘤双模诊断及热休克抑制的光热治疗

成功地发生了反应(图4-7(b))。iRGD-$W_{18}O_{49}$纳米颗粒(图4-7(c))和$W_{18}O_{49}$-17AAG纳米颗粒(图4-7(d))的傅里叶变换红外光谱结果显示出相同的趋势。

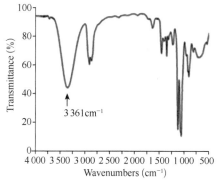

(a) $W_{18}O_{49}$纳米颗粒的傅里叶变换红外光谱结果

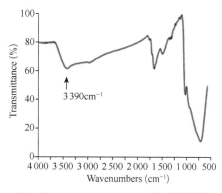

(b) iRGD-$W_{18}O_{49}$-17AAG纳米颗粒的傅里叶变换红外光谱结果

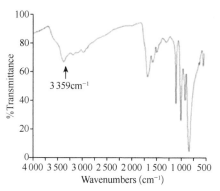

(c) iRGD-$W_{18}O_{49}$纳米颗粒的傅里叶变换红外光谱结果

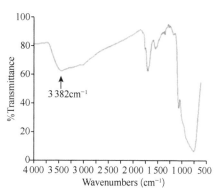

(d) $W_{18}O_{49}$-17AAG纳米颗粒的傅里叶变换红外光谱结果

图4-7 不同纳米颗粒的傅里叶变换红外光谱结果

图片来自参考文献[60]

此外,测定了溶解在DMSO中的不同浓度梯度下17AAG的紫外-可见-近红外光谱结果(图4-8(a))。使用紫外-可见-近红外光谱中320 nm波长下的吸收值绘制了17AAG的标准浓度曲线。如图4-8(b)所示,17AAG的吸光度随着其浓度的增加而增加,且二者之间存在明显的线性关系,证实了可通过UV-vis-NIR结果验证纳米颗粒中装载17AAG的浓度。

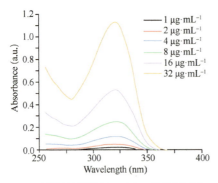
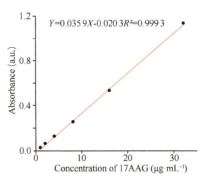

(a) 不同浓度梯度 17AAG 的紫外-可见-近红外光谱结果

(b) 不同浓度梯度 17AAG 的在 320 nm 波长下的紫外-可见-近红外光吸收强度

图 4-8　17AAG 的紫外-可见-近红外光谱结果

图片来自参考文献[60]

最后,验证了 iRGD-$W_{18}O_{49}$-17AAG 纳米颗粒的光热治疗能力。如图 4-9(a) 所示,在使用 808 nm 激光(2 W·cm^{-2})照射 5 min 后,$W_{18}O_{49}$ 纳米颗粒悬浮液的温度由 20.7 ℃上升到 44.3 ℃,iRGD-$W_{18}O_{49}$-17AAG 纳米颗粒悬浮液的温度由 20.1 ℃上升到 41.9 ℃。然而,PBS 中只观察到了温度的轻微升高(从 20.4 ℃上升至 21.8 ℃)。这些结果证实此纳米颗粒具有可靠的光热治疗性能。同时,如图 4-9(b)所示,iRGD-$W_{18}O_{49}$-17AAG 纳米颗粒可在 PBS 及血清中保持至少 50 h 稳定的水合粒径,表明其具有较好的稳定性。

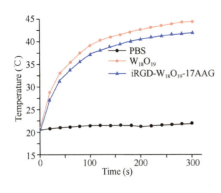
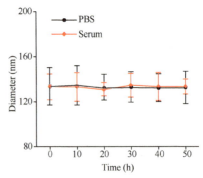

(a) 808 nm 激光照射下不同纳米颗粒的温度随时间变化的曲线

(b) 每 10 h 的水合粒径结果

图 4-9　iRGD-$W_{18}O_{49}$-17AAG 纳米颗粒的光热治疗能力结果

图片来自参考文献[60]

4.3.2 胃肠道恶性肿瘤细胞的选择性摄取

根据既往的研究,胃肠道恶性肿瘤细胞表达高水平的整合素 $\alpha_v\beta_3$ 受体,而正常胃上皮细胞 GES-1 表达低水平的整合素 $\alpha_v\beta_3$ 受体[58-59]。为了证实 iRGD-$W_{18}O_{49}$-17AAG 纳米颗粒在胃肠道恶性肿瘤细胞中的选择性摄取,使用 Cy5.5 修饰纳米颗粒,并且以 GES-1 细胞作为对照组。如图 4-10(a)所示,使用 iRGD-$W_{18}O_{49}$-17AAG 纳米颗粒共培养后,MKN-45P 细胞内可见明显的荧光信号,而 GES-1 细胞内仅可检测到微弱的荧光信号。而未与纳米颗粒共培养的组,MKN-45P 细胞和 GES-1 细胞内均几乎检测不到荧光(图 4-10(b))。以上结果证实了在连接了 iRGD 后,纳米颗粒可以显著增强其被胃肠道恶性肿瘤细胞主动摄取的能力。

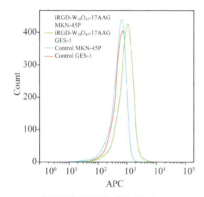

(a) 胃肠道恶性肿瘤细胞和 GES-1 胃上皮细胞分别与 iRGD-$W_{18}O_{49}$-17AAG 纳米颗粒和 PBS 共培养后的流式细胞术结果

(b) 不同组别流式细胞术中的平均荧光强度

数据以平均值±标准差表示,*** 代表 $p<0.001$。

图 4-10 胃肠道恶性肿瘤细胞对于 iRGD-$W_{18}O_{49}$-17AAG 纳米颗粒的选择性摄取

图片来自参考文献[60]

4.3.3 体内生物分布及活体近红外荧光成像

为确定两种纳米颗粒在体内的生物分布,采用 ICP-MS 法测定肿瘤组织和主要脏器中钨的含量。如图 4-11 所示,注射后 24 h,iRGD-$W_{18}O_{49}$-17AAG 组肿瘤组织的钨含量达到峰值,是 $W_{18}O_{49}$ 组的 5 倍。同时也测定了注射后 1 h、4 h、12 h 和 48 h 各组织的钨含量。有趣的是,无论在任何时间点,iRGD-$W_{18}O_{49}$-17AAG 组肿瘤组织的钨含量均大于 $W_{18}O_{49}$ 组,而肝脏和脾脏组织的钨含量则更少。以上结果可以证明 iRGD-$W_{18}O_{49}$-17AAG 纳米颗粒具有良好的生物相容性,且可有效地防止自体的免疫清除,进而降低对其他器官的非特异性毒性。

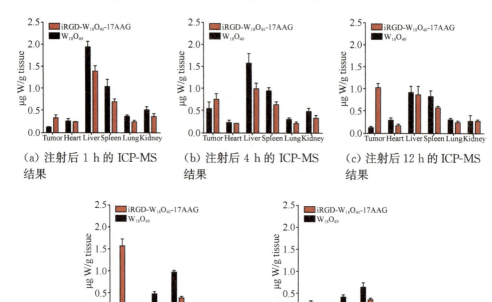

(a) 注射后 1 h 的 ICP-MS 结果

(b) 注射后 4 h 的 ICP-MS 结果

(c) 注射后 12 h 的 ICP-MS 结果

(d) 注射后 24 h 的 ICP-MS 结果

(e) 注射后 48 h 的 ICP-MS 结果

注射量为每只小鼠 100 μL(钨 1 mg/mL)。数据以平均值±标准差表示。

图 4-11 注射后不同时间点 $W_{18}O_{49}$ 和 iRGD-$W_{18}O_{49}$-17AAG 纳米颗粒的体内生物分布

图片来自参考文献[60]

之后,使用 Cy5.5 修饰 iRGD-$W_{18}O_{49}$-17AAG 纳米颗粒,进一步证实其在体内对于肿瘤的蓄积。尾静脉注射 iRGD-$W_{18}O_{49}$-17AAG 纳米颗粒后,使用实时活体荧光成像系统在不同时间点采集实时近红外成像结果。用不同的颜色显示不同的荧光强度,荧光强度按红、黄、绿、蓝的顺序递减。如图 4-12(a)所示,荧光信号在注射后 4 h 可在肿瘤区域观察到,且随着时间的推移荧光强度逐渐增强。而注射 1 h 后肝区可见明显的荧光信号,提示纳米颗粒可被网状内皮系统快速识别。与 ICP-MS 结果一致,注射后 24 h 在肿瘤组织中检测到最强的荧光信号。尾静脉注射 24 h 后心、肝、脾、肺、肾和肿瘤组织的离体近红外荧光图像也证明了肿瘤组织具有很强烈的荧光(图 4-12(b))。如图 4-12(c)所示,肿瘤组织的荧光信号强度高于任何器官。以上结果可以证明 iRGD-$W_{18}O_{49}$-17AAG 纳米颗粒具有良好的

第 4 章 主动靶向性氧化钨纳米颗粒介导的胃肠道恶性肿瘤双模诊断及热休克抑制的光热治疗

生物相容性,且可有效地防止自体的免疫清除,能有效地蓄积至胃肠道恶性肿瘤病灶中,与体外细胞结果表现出了相似的肿瘤靶向性,进而发挥胃肠道恶性肿瘤主动靶向性的诊断与治疗相结合功能。

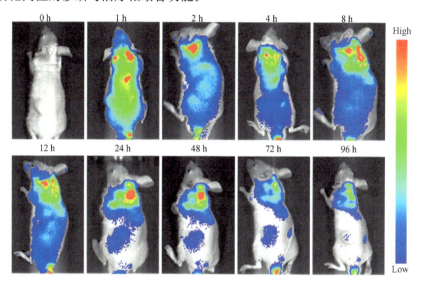

(a) 尾静脉注射 iRGD-$W_{18}O_{49}$-17AAG 纳米颗粒后不同时间点胃肠道恶性肿瘤异位移植瘤小鼠的实时活体近红外荧光图像

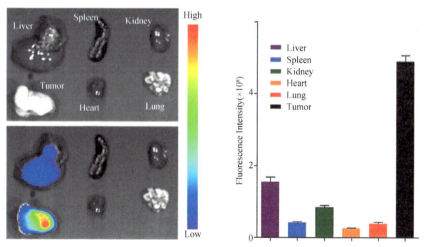

(b) 尾静脉注射 24 h 后心、肝、脾、肺、肾和肿瘤组织的离体白光和近红外荧光图像

(c) 尾静脉注射 24 h 后心、肝、脾、肺、肾和肿瘤组织的离体荧光信号强度

数据以平均值±标准差表示。

图 4-12 iRGD-$W_{18}O_{49}$-17AAG 的活体近红外荧光成像

图片来自参考文献[60]

4.3.4 体外 CT 成像结果

三维的 CT 成像由于能够清晰地显示临床特征和解剖细节,在临床上得到了广泛的应用。同时,由于 $W_{18}O_{49}$ 纳米颗粒具有很强的吸收 X 射线的能力,其有望成为令临床满意的 CT 造影剂。首先,测定 iRGD-$W_{18}O_{49}$-17AAG 纳米颗粒的体外 CT 特性。首先测量 iRGD-$W_{18}O_{49}$-17AAG 纳米颗粒和临床上最常用的 CT 增强扫描造影剂碘丙醇的体外 CT 图像。如图 4-13(a)所示,在相同的碘和钨浓度下,iRGD-$W_{18}O_{49}$-17AAG 纳米颗粒的 CT 值明显高于碘丙醇。同时,其亨氏单位(Hounsfield Unit,HU)值与钨的浓度呈良好的相关线性关系(图 4-13(b)),并且其斜率(12.974)明显高于碘丙醇的斜率(3.284)。以上结果证实了 iRGD-$W_{18}O_{49}$-17AAG 纳米颗粒具有良好的体外 CT 成像效果。

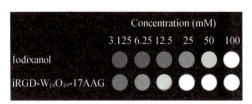

(a) 不同碘和钨浓度的碘丙醇和 iRGD-$W_{18}O_{49}$-17AAG 纳米颗粒的 CT 图像

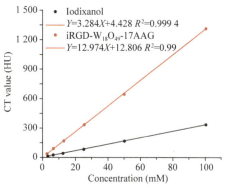

(b) 碘和钨浓度与 CT 值的关系

图 4-13 iRGD-$W_{18}O_{49}$-17AAG 纳米颗粒的体外 CT 成像结果

图片来自参考文献[60]

4.3.5 小鼠体内 CT 成像结果

在证实了 iRGD-$W_{18}O_{49}$-17AAG 纳米颗粒具有良好的体外 CT 成像效果之后,采用 MKN-45P 异位移植瘤模型进一步检测其体内 CT 成像的效果。根据体内生物分布和活体近红外荧光成像结果,选择注射后的 24 h 作为研究时间点。经过海斯菲德重建软件分析和重建,结果如图 4-14 所示。在注射碘丙醇后,由于快速的肾脏代谢,几乎没有药物富集到肿瘤区域。相比之下,尾静脉注射 iRGD-$W_{18}O_{49}$-17AAG 纳米颗粒后 24 h 的小鼠肿瘤部位的亮度达到峰值,同时肿瘤组织轮廓清晰(白色箭头)。这些结果进一步证明了 iRGD-$W_{18}O_{49}$-17AAG 纳米颗粒能有效地积聚到肿瘤组织中,表现出了优越的肿瘤主动靶向性。

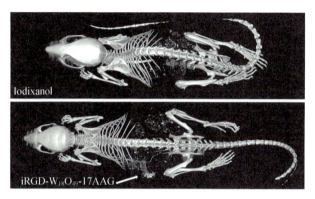

肿瘤组织用白色箭头指出。

图 4-14 尾静脉注射碘丙醇和 iRGD-W$_{18}$O$_{49}$-17AAG 纳米颗粒后 24 h 的小鼠体内 CT 成像结果

图片来自参考文献[60]

4.3.6 体外红外热成像结果

之后,利用红外热像仪研究了 iRGD-W$_{18}$O$_{49}$-17AAG 纳米颗粒的体外光热治疗性质。如图 4-15 所示,当固定钨浓度为 100 μg/mL 时,纳米颗粒溶液的温度在强度为 2 W·cm^{-2} 的 808 nm 激光下照射 5 min 后,温度迅速从 33.6 ℃ 升高到 44.3 ℃。以上结果证实了 iRGD-W$_{18}$O$_{49}$-17AAG 纳米颗粒具有良好的体外光热能力。

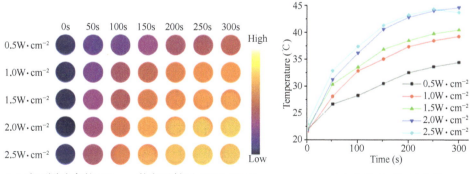

(a) 在不同功率的 808 nm 激光照射下,iRGD-W$_{18}$O$_{49}$-17AAG 纳米颗粒在 PBS 中的红外热成像结果

(b) 温度曲线随时间的变化

图 4-15 iRGD-W$_{18}$O$_{49}$-17AAG 纳米颗粒的体外红外热成像结果

图片来自参考文献[60]

4.3.7 小鼠体内红外热成像结果

根据体外结果,确定了 808 nm 激光的照射参数为 5 min、2 W·cm^{-2}。在照射后,iRGD-$W_{18}O_{49}$-17AAG 组的小鼠肿瘤区域的温度从 32.2 ℃ 上升到 43.2 ℃ (图 4-16)。相比之下,iRGD-$W_{18}O_{49}$ 组和 $W_{18}O_{49}$-17AAG 组小鼠肿瘤区域的温度也表现了一定的增加,但低于 iRGD-$W_{18}O_{49}$-17AAG 组。PBS 对照组小鼠肿瘤区域的温度增长缓慢,从 30.6 ℃ 上升到 34.7 ℃。结果表明,iRGD-$W_{18}O_{49}$-17AAG 纳米颗粒可以有效地靶向肿瘤组织并抑制肿瘤的热阻抗,进而在 808 nm 激光的照射可以使肿瘤部位温度显著升高,达到了有效的光热治疗效果。

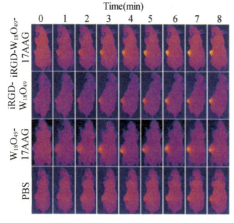

(a) 不同纳米颗粒尾静脉注射后 MKN-45P 异位移植瘤模型的活体红外热成像图

(b) 不同纳米颗粒组肿瘤区域的温度时间曲线

图 4-16　不同治疗后小鼠的体内红外热成像结果

图片来自参考文献[60]

4.3.8 体外抗肿瘤治疗效果

在证实了 iRGD-$W_{18}O_{49}$-17AAG 纳米颗粒在体内外的肿瘤主动靶向能力后,进一步研究了不同组的细胞毒性。使用 CCK-8 法和 Calcein-AM/PI 双染法观察这种热休克抑制的增强光热治疗对于 MKN-45P 细胞的杀伤作用。如图 4-17(a)所示,对照、激光照射和 iRGD-$W_{18}O_{49}$-17AAG 组的胃肠道恶性肿瘤细胞未表现出明显的细胞毒性。$W_{18}O_{49}$-17AAG+激光照射组的细胞表现出中等的活力,而 iRGD-$W_{18}O_{49}$-17AAG+激光照射组表现出强烈的细胞杀伤作用,MKN-45P 细胞约为对照组的 30%。以上结果证实了在引入 iRGD 后,纳米颗粒可以在靶向整合素 $\alpha_v\beta_3$ 受体后,通过细胞介导的内吞作用选择性地聚集到

第 4 章 主动靶向性氧化钨纳米颗粒介导的胃肠道恶性肿瘤双模诊断及热休克抑制的光热治疗

胃肠道恶性肿瘤细胞中,并在 808 nm 激光照射下更有效地杀死细胞。此外,iRGD-$W_{18}O_{49}$+激光照射组和 iRGD-$W_{18}O_{49}$-17AAG+激光照射组的细胞活力存在显著性的差异(**)。这一有趣的现象可能主要是由于 HSP90 的过度表达可能被特异性地抑制,从而使得 $W_{18}O_{49}$ 的光热治疗效果得到了有效的增强。之后,使用 Calcein-AM/PI 双染法进一步检测不同组细胞的活力。如图 4-17(b)所示,iRGD-$W_{18}O_{49}$-17AAG+激光照射组可观察到最多的死细胞,而 $W_{18}O_{49}$-17AAG+激光照射组和 iRGD-$W_{18}O_{49}$+激光照射组可观察到中等量的死细胞。以上结果表明,iRGD-$W_{18}O_{49}$-17AAG 纳米颗粒在体外具有较好的生物安全性,同时可在 808 nm 激光的照射下,对于 MKN-45P 细胞具有较强的光热治疗作用,可进一步用于体内的肿瘤治疗。

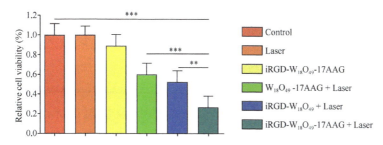

(a) 使用 CCK-8 试剂盒测定不同处理后的细胞活力

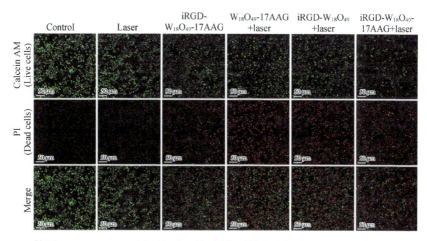

(b) 使用 Calcein-AM/PI 活死细胞双染试剂盒拍摄不同处理后细胞的 CLSM 图像

绿色荧光表示活细胞,红色荧光表示死细胞,标尺是 50 μm。数据以平均值±标准差表示,** 代表 $p<0.01$;*** 代表 $p<0.001$。

图 4-17 不同处理后细胞毒性的检测

图片来自参考文献[60]

4.3.9 体内抗肿瘤治疗效果

首先,将 MKN-45P 异位移植瘤小鼠随机分为 6 组,观察其对于体内光热治疗的疗效。如图 4-18(a)所示,激光照射组对肿瘤的生长几乎没有抑制作用,而 iRGD-$W_{18}O_{49}$-17AAG 组对肿瘤有轻微的抗肿瘤作用。相比之下,iRGD-$W_{18}O_{49}$+激光照射组和 $W_{18}O_{49}$-17AAG+激光照射组的肿瘤生长受到了中度的抑制。有趣的是,iRGD-$W_{18}O_{49}$-17AAG+激光照射组的小鼠肿瘤体积在前 6 天生长缓慢,而在第 6 天后体积开始减小。上述结果证实了 iRGD-$W_{18}O_{49}$-17AAG 介导的光热治疗在体内具有良好的治疗效果。与肿瘤体积的变化相比,第 16 天从小鼠体内采集到肿瘤组织的图像和重量均表现出类似的肿瘤体积变化趋势(图 4-18(b)、(c))。之后,进一步用肿瘤组织的 H-E 和 TUNEL 染色研究不同治疗组的光热治疗疗效。H-E 切片显示,在 iRGD-$W_{18}O_{49}$-17AAG+激光照射组中,大多数肿瘤细胞被严重破坏,如核破裂、核固缩和核溶解(图 4-18(d))。此外,iRGD-$W_{18}O_{49}$+激光照射组的肿瘤细胞损伤明显多于 $W_{18}O_{49}$-17AAG+激光照射组,证实了 iRGD-$W_{18}O_{49}$-17AAG 纳米颗粒可达到最优越的光热治疗效果。TUNEL 切片中代表凋亡的暗褐色细胞核表现出了类似的结果。因此,我们使用这种方法来观察各个治疗组的肿瘤组织切片的凋亡情况。有趣的是,TUNEL 染色结果显示出了与 H-E 切片相似的趋势,这表明纳米颗粒的光热治疗效果随着整合素靶向多肽(iRGD)和 HSP90 抑制剂(17AAG)的连接而取得了更好的疗效。综上所述,我们可以认为 iRGD-$W_{18}O_{49}$-17AAG 纳米颗粒在接受 808 nm 激光(2 W·cm^{-2})照射后,在诱导胃肠道恶性肿瘤细胞凋亡和坏死方面表现最好,并表现出了体内良好的抑制肿瘤组织生长的效果。

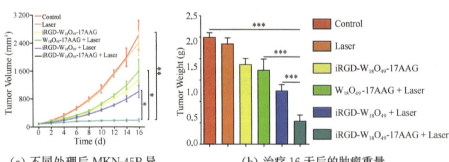

(a) 不同处理后 MKN-45P 异种移植瘤小鼠治疗 16 天后的体重曲线

(b) 治疗 16 天后的肿瘤重量

第4章 主动靶向性氧化钨纳米颗粒介导的胃肠道恶性肿瘤双模诊断及热休克抑制的光热治疗

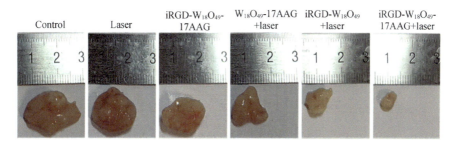

(c) 治疗16天后的肿瘤照片

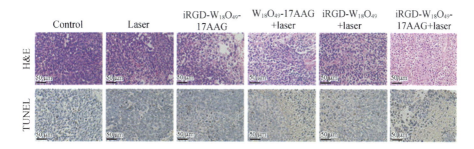

(d) 治疗16天后肿瘤组织的H-E和TUNEL染色结果,标尺是50 μm

数据以平均值±标准差表示,*代表$p<0.05$;**代表$p<0.01$;***代表$p<0.001$。

图4-18 不同治疗后体内抗肿瘤治疗效果检测

图片来自参考文献[60]

4.3.10 生物安全分析

为了评估纳米颗粒的体内生物安全性,在不同的治疗的过程中,监测小鼠体重,期间几乎没有发现体重存在波动(图4-19(a))。同时,结束后收集了小鼠血液进行血生化和血液学(图4-19(b))分析,评估其潜在细胞毒性。各组的肝功能(ALT、AST)、肾功能(BUN、Scr)、免疫应答反应(WBC、NEU、LYM)、细胞毒性(RBC、HGB)和脾功能(PLT)结果均未存在显著性差异。最后,收集小鼠的心、肝、脾、肺和肾进行H-E染色。如图4-19(c)所示,所有组均表现出可忽略的炎症损伤、组织学异常以及坏死。以上结果表明iRGD-$W_{18}O_{49}$-17AAG纳米颗粒治疗时具有很高的生物安全性,主要原因可能是由于肿瘤主动靶向性给药,降低了对非肿瘤器官的副作用。

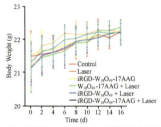
(a) 治疗16天的小鼠体重曲线

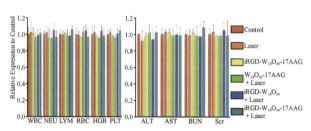
(b) 治疗16天后的血液学检查及血清生化学检查,包括白细胞(WBC)、中性粒细胞(NEU)、淋巴细胞(LYM)、红细胞(RBC)、血红蛋白(HGB)、血小板(PLT)、谷丙转氨酶(ALT)、谷草转氨酶(AST)、血尿素氮(BUN)和血肌酐(Scr)

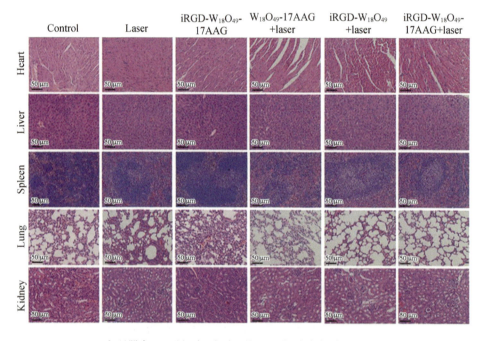
(c) 主要器官(心、肝、脾、肺、肾)的H-E切片染色,标尺是50 μm

数据以平均值±标准差表示。

图4-19　不同治疗后体内生物安全性分析

图片来自参考文献[60]

4.4 结果与讨论

综上所述,首次成功地合成了一种新型的纳米颗粒,通过同时实现在808 nm的激光照射下的肿瘤主动靶向、热休克反应抑制的光热治疗以及CT/

第4章 主动靶向性氧化钨纳米颗粒介导的胃肠道恶性肿瘤双模诊断及热休克抑制的光热治疗

NIR 荧光双模下的疗效监测从而更有效地诊断和治疗胃肠道恶性肿瘤。其中，$W_{18}O_{49}$ 纳米颗粒由于具有较高的光热性能和吸收 X 射线的能力，且存在较多的活性基团，可被用作纳米载体。而 iRGD 作为一种新型的环状多肽被进一步结合到纳米载体上，从而使其更有效地穿透胃肠道恶性肿瘤细胞。同时，iRGD-$W_{18}O_{49}$-17AAG 纳米颗粒具有热休克抑制的能力，进而抵抗肿瘤组织的热保护作用，增强光热治疗的疗效，可有效抑制肿瘤生长。此外，iRGD-$W_{18}O_{49}$-17AAG 纳米颗粒在体外和体内的生物安全性评价方面也初步显示出强烈的优越性。同时，这种纳米颗粒由于其自身可作为 CT 和近红外荧光成像的造影剂，可诊断肿瘤的发生并监测治疗效果。这是首次以 $W_{18}O_{49}$ 纳米颗粒为核心，通过抑制热休克反应来克服肿瘤组织的耐热性，进而增强 808 nm 激光照射下光热治疗的效果。总之，在 CT/NIR 荧光双模成像的指导下，iRGD-$W_{18}O_{49}$-17AAG 可以在肿瘤组织中聚集，进而穿透癌细胞，抑制热休克反应，从而增强光热治疗的效果，实现对恶性肿瘤组织的精准消融。我们的工作为肿瘤主动靶向、热休克反应抑制和双模监测/指导光热治疗的疗效提供了新的方向[60]。

参考文献

[1] ISOBE Y, NASHIMOTO A, AKAZAWA K, et al. Gastric cancer treatment in Japan: 2008 annual report of the JGCA nationwide registry. Gastric Cancer, 2011, 14(4): 301-316.

[2] ALLEMANI C, WEIR H K, CARREIRA H, et al. Global surveillance of cancer survival 1995—2009: analysis of individual data for 25 676 887 patients from 279 population-based registries in 67 countries (CONCORD-2). Lancet, 2015, 385(9972): 977-1010.

[3] SHI H, SUN Y, YAN R, et al. Magnetic semiconductor Gd-doping CuS nanoparticles as activatable nanoprobes for bimodal imaging and targeted photothermal therapy of gastric tumors. Nano Lett., 2019, 19(2): 937-947.

[4] Bray F, Ferlay J, Soerjomataram I, et al. Global cancer statistics 2018: GLOBOCAN estimates of incidence and mortality worldwide for 36 cancers in 185 countries. CA Cancer J Clin., 2018, 68(6): 394-424.

[5] VAN CUTSEM E, SAGAERT X, TOPAL B, et al. Gastric cancer. Lancet, 2016, 388(10060): 2654-2664.

[6] CHEN W, ZHENG R, BAADE P D, et al. Cancer statistics in China, 2015. CA Cancer J Clin., 2016, 66(2):115-132.

[7] Ko K P, Shin A, Cho S, et al. Environmental contributions to gastrointestinal and liver cancer in the Asia-Pacific region. J Gastroenterol Hepatol., 2018, 33(1):111-120.

[8] ZHANG X, WANG S, WANG H, et al. Circular RNA circNRIP1 acts as a microRNA-149-5p sponge to promote gastric cancer progression via the AKT1/mTOR pathway. Mol Cancer., 2019, 18(1):20.

[9] CHENG L, WANG C, FENG L, et al. Functional nanomaterials for phototherapies of cancer. Chem Rev., 2014, 114(21):10869-10939.

[10] CUI M, TANG D, WANG B, et al. Bioorthogonal guided activation of cGAS-STING by AIE photosensitizer nanoparticles for targeted tumor therapy and imaging. Adv Mater., 2023, 35(52):e2305668.

[11] SHI H, YAN R, WU L, et al. Tumor-targeting CuS nanoparticles for multimodal imaging and guided photothermal therapy of lymph node metastasis. Acta Biomater, 2018, 72:256-265.

[12] ZHENG B, BAI Y, CHEN H, et al. Targeted delivery of tungsten oxide nanoparticles for multifunctional anti-tumor therapy via macrophages. Biomater Sci., 2018, 6(6):1379-1389.

[13] LI H, WANG K, YANG X, et al. Dual-function nanostructured lipid carriers to deliver IR780 for breast cancer treatment: anti-metastatic and photothermal anti-tumor therapy. Acta Biomater, 2017, 53:399-413.

[14] YANG Y, ZHU W, DONG Z, et al. 1D coordination polymer nanofibers for low-temperature photothermal therapy. Adv Mater., 2017, 29(40):201703588.

[15] SHANMUGAM V, SELVAKUMAR S, YEH C S. Near-infrared light-responsive nanomaterials in cancer therapeutics. Chem Soc Rev., 2014, 43(17):6254-6287.

[16] REN S, CHENG X, CHEN M, et al. Hypotoxic and rapidly metabolic PEG-PCL-C3-ICG nanoparticles for fluorescence-guided photothermal/photodynamic therapy against OSCC. ACS Appl Mater Interfaces.,

2017,9(37):31509-31518.

[17] CHEN M,TANG S,GUO Z,et al. Core-shell Pd@Au nanoplates as theranostic agents for in-vivo photoacoustic imaging, CT imaging, and photothermal therapy. Adv Mater. ,2014,26(48):8210-8216.

[18] YANG K,FENG L,SHI X,et al. Nano-graphene in biomedicine: theranostic applications. Chem Soc Rev. ,2013,42(2):530-547.

[19] LEE S B,YOON G,LEE S W,et al. Combined positron emission tomography and cerenkov luminescence imaging of sentinel lymph nodes using PEGylated radionuclide-embedded gold nanoparticles. Small, 2016,12(35):4894-4901.

[20] ZHANG M K,WANG X G,ZHU J Y,et al. Double-targeting explosible nanofirework for tumor ignition to guide tumor-depth photothermal therapy. Small,2018,14(20):e1800292.

[21] ZHU A,MIAO K,DENG Y,et al. dually pH/reduction-responsive vesicles for ultrahigh-contrast fluorescence imaging and thermo-chemotherapy-synergized tumor ablation. ACS Nano. ,2015,9(8):7874-7885.

[22] GUO M,MAO H,LI Y,et al. Dual imaging-guided photothermal/photodynamic therapy using micelles. Biomaterials,2014,35(16):4656-4666.

[23] JAQUE D,MARTÍNEZ MAESTRO L,DEL ROSAL B,et al. Nanoparticles for photothermal therapies. Nanoscale,2014,6(16):9494-9530.

[24] TIAN T,ZHANG H X,HE C P,et al. Surface functionalized exosomes as targeted drug delivery vehicles for cerebral ischemia therapy. Biomaterials,2018,150:137-149.

[25] TAVEIRA-DASILVA A M,JONES A M,JULIEN-WILLIAMS P,et al. Long-term effect of Sirolimus on serum vascular endothelial growth factor D levels in patients with lymphangioleiomyomatosis. Chest. ,2018, 153(1):124-132.

[26] Elzoghby A O,Mostafa S K,Helmy M W,et al. Superiority of aromatase inhibitor and cyclooxygenase-2 inhibitor combined delivery: Hyaluronate-targeted versus PEGylated protamine nanocapsules for breast cancer therapy. Int J Pharm. ,2017,529(1-2):178-192.

[27] GOETZ M P, TOI M, CAMPONE M, et al. MONARCH 3: Abemaciclib as initial therapy for advanced breast cancer. J Clin Oncol., 2017, 35(32): 3638-3646.

[28] DING N, ZOU Z, SHA H, et al. iRGD synergizes with PD-1 knockout immunotherapy by enhancing lymphocyte infiltration in gastric cancer. Nat Commun., 2019, 10(1): 1336.

[29] SPARANO J A, GRAY R J, MAKOWER D F, et al. Adjuvant Chemotherapy Guided by a 21-Gene expression assay in breast cancer. N Engl J Med., 2018, 379(2): 111-121.

[30] HAMBLEY T W, HAIT W N. Is anticancer drug development heading in the right direction? Cancer Res., 2009, 69(4): 1259-1262.

[31] MINCHINTON A I, TANNOCK I F. Drug penetration in solid tumours. Nat Rev Cancer., 2006, 6(8): 583-592.

[32] DIAZ BESSONE M I, SIMÓN-GRACIA L, SCODELLER P, et al. iRGD-guided tamoxifen polymersomes inhibit estrogen receptor transcriptional activity and decrease the number of breast cancer cells with self-renewing capacity. J Nanobiotechnology., 2019, 17(1): 120.

[33] AI S, ZHEN S, LIU Z, et al. An iRGD peptide conjugated heparin nanocarrier for gastric cancer therapy. RSC Adv., 2018, 8(52): 30012-30020.

[34] SUGAHARA K N, TEESALU T, KARMALI P P, et al. Tissue-penetrating delivery of compounds and nanoparticles into tumors. Cancer Cell, 2009, 16(6): 510-520.

[35] SUGAHARA K N, TEESALU T, KARMALI P P, et al. Coadministration of a tumor-penetrating peptide enhances the efficacy of cancer drugs. Science, 2010, 328(5981): 1031-1035.

[36] FISHER J W, SARKAR S, BUCHANAN C F, et al. Photothermal response of human and murine cancer cells to multiwalled carbon nanotubes after laser irradiation. Cancer Res., 2010, 70(23): 9855-9864.

[37] RYBINSKI M, SZYMANSKA Z, LASOTA S, et al. Modelling the efficacy of hyperthermia treatment. J R Soc Interface., 2013, 10(88): 20130527.

[38] LEE S W, LEE J W, CHUNG J H, et al. Expression of heat shock protein 27

in prostate cancer cell lines according to the extent of malignancy and doxazosin treatment. World J Mens Health., 2013,31(3):247-253.

[39] FRAZIER N, PAYNE A, DILLON C, et al. Enhanced efficacy of combination heat shock targeted polymer therapeutics with high intensity focused ultrasound. Nanomedicine, 2017,13(3):1235-1243.

[40] WANG L, HUNT K E, MARTIN G M, et al. Structure and function of the human Werner syndrome gene promoter: evidence for transcriptional modulation. Nucleic Acids Res., 1998,26(15):3480-3485.

[41] NEWMAN B, LIU Y, LEE H F, et al. HSP90 inhibitor 17-AAG selectively eradicates lymphoma stem cells. Cancer Res., 2012,72(17):4551-4561.

[42] ZHANG J, ZHENG Z, ZHAO Y, et al. The heat shock protein 90 inhibitor 17-AAG suppresses growth and induces apoptosis in human cholangiocarcinoma cells. Clin Exp Med., 2013,13(4):323-328.

[43] ZHANG L, WANG D, YANG K, et al. Mitochondria-targeted artificial "Nano-RBCs" for amplified synergistic cancer phototherapy by a single NIR irradiation. Adv Sci(Weinh)., 2018,5(8):1800049.

[44] DE FATIMA VASCO ARAGAO M, VAN DER LINDEN V, BRAINER-LIMA A M, et al. Clinical features and neuroimaging (CT and MRI) findings in presumed Zika virus related congenital infection and microcephaly: retrospective case series study. BMJ., 2016,353:i1901.

[45] HUANG Y Q, LIANG C H, HE L, et al. Development and validation of a radiomics Nomogram for preoperative prediction of lymph node metastasis in colorectal cancer. J Clin Oncol., 2016,34(18):2157-2164.

[46] LIU Y, LI L, GUO Q, et al. Novel Cs-based upconversion nanoparticles as dual-modal CT and UCL imaging agents for chemo-photothermal synergistic therapy. Theranostics, 2016,6(10):1491-1505.

[47] WANG G, QIAN K, MEI X. A theranostic nanoplatform: magneto-gold @fluorescence polymer nanoparticles for tumor targeting T_1 & T_2-MRI/CT/NIR fluorescence imaging and induction of genuine autophagy mediated chemotherapy. Nanoscale, 2018,10(22):10467-10478.

[48] He H, Lin Y, Tian Z Q, et al. Ultrasmall Pb:Ag$_2$S quantum dots with uniform particle size and bright tunable fluorescence in the NIR-II window. Small, 2018, 14(11): e1703296.

[49] LI X, SCHUMANN C, ALBARQI H A, et al. A tumor-activatable theranostic nanomedicine platform for NIR fluorescence-guided surgery and combinatorial phototherapy. Theranostics, 2018, 8(3): 767 – 784.

[50] ZHAO P, REN S, LIU Y, et al. PL-W$_{18}$O$_{49}$-TPZ nanoparticles for simultaneous hypoxia-activated chemotherapy and photothermal therapy. ACS Appl Mater Interfaces., 2018, 10(4): 3405 – 3413.

[51] HUO D, DING J, CUI Y X, et al. X-ray CT and pneumonia inhibition properties of gold-silver nanoparticles for targeting MRSA induced pneumonia. Biomaterials, 2014, 35(25): 7032 – 7041.

[52] HUO D, HE J, LI H, et al. X-ray CT guided fault-free photothermal ablation of metastatic lymph nodes with ultrafine HER-2 targeting W18O49 nanoparticles. Biomaterials, 2014, 35(33): 9155 – 9166.

[53] YANG B, JIN S, GUO S, et al. Recent development of SERS technology: semiconductor-based study. ACS Omega., 2019, 4(23): 20101 – 20108.

[54] WANG Y, SHANG W, NIU M, et al. Hypoxia-active nanoparticles used in tumor theranostic. Int J Nanomedicine., 2019, 14: 3705 – 3722.

[55] LI Y, LIAN Y, ZHANG L T, et al. Cell and nanoparticle transport in tumour microvasculature: the role of size, shape and surface functionality of nanoparticles. Interface Focus, 2016, 6(1): 20150086.

[56] NIE S. Understanding and overcoming major barriers in cancer nanomedicine. Nanomedicine(Lond), 2010, 5(4): 523 – 528.

[57] Liu Y, Tan J, Thomas A, et al. The shape of things to come: importance of design in nanotechnology for drug delivery. Ther Deliv., 2012, 3(2): 181 – 194.

[58] SIMÓN-GRACIA L, HUNT H, TEESALU T. Peritoneal carcinomatosis targeting with tumor homing peptides. Molecules, 2018, 23(5): 1190.

[59] ZHU A, SHA H, SU S, et al. Bispecific tumor-penetrating protein anti-EGFR-iRGD efficiently enhances the infiltration of lymphocytes in gas-

tric cancer. Am J Cancer Res., 2018,8(1):91-105.

[60] Yang Z, Wang J, Liu S, et al. Tumor-targeting $W_{18}O_{49}$ nanoparticles for dual-modality imaging and guided heat-shock-response-inhibited photothermal therapy in gastric cancer. Particle & Particle Systems Characterization, 2019,36:1900124.

附录

主要缩略词表

英文缩写	英文全称	中文全称
CT	Computed Tomography	计算机断层扫描
MRI	Magnetic Resonance Imaging	磁共振成像
PET-CT	Positron Emission Computed Tomography	正电子发射计算机断层扫描
EPR	Enhanced Permeability and Retention	高通透性和滞留
GNPs	Gold Nanoparticles	金纳米粒子
FA	Folic acid	叶酸
GSH	Glutathione	谷胱甘肽
MMP	Matrix Metalloproteinase	基质金属蛋白酶
PEG	Polyethylene Glycol	聚乙二醇
HER-2	Human Epidermal Growth Factor Receptor-2	人表皮生长因子受体2
FDA	Food and Drug Administration	食品和药物管理局
NIR	Near-Infrared	近红外
ICG	Indocyanine Green	吲哚菁绿
PBS	Phosphate Buffered Saline	磷酸盐缓冲液
FBS	Fetal Bovine Serum	胎牛血清
CA125	Carbohydrate Antigen 125	糖类抗原125
CEA	Carcinoembryonic Antigen	癌胚抗原
CTCs	Circulating Tumor Cells	循环肿瘤细胞
PS	Performance Status	功能状态评分
PCI	Peritoneal Cancer Index	腹膜癌指数
MSNs	Mesoporous Silica Nanoparticles	介孔二氧化硅纳米粒
ROS	Reactive Oxygen Species	活性氧
PCL	Polycaprolactone	聚己内酯
MET	Metformin	二甲双胍
PDT	Photodynamic Therapy	光动力疗法
PTT	Photothermal Therapy	光热疗法

续表

英文缩写	英文全称	中文全称
PA	Photoacoustic	光声
HSP90	Heat Shock Protein 90	热休克蛋白 90
17AAG	Tanespimycin	坦螺旋霉素
DMSO	Dimethyl Sulfoxide	二甲基亚砜
CLSM	Confocal Laser Scanning Microscope	激光共聚焦扫描显微镜
TEM	Transmission Electron Microscopy	透射电子显微镜
SEM	Scanning Electron Microscopy	场发射扫描电子显微镜
DLS	Dynamic Light Scattering	动态光散射
XRD	X-ray Diffraction	X 射线衍射
XPS	X-ray Photoelectron Spectroscopy	X 射线光电子能谱
FTIR	Fourier Transform Infrared	傅里叶变换红外光谱
UV-vis-NIR	Ultraviolet-visible-Near-Infrared	紫外-可见-近红外
HIF-1α	Hypoxia Inducible Factor-1α	缺氧诱导因子-1α
PVDF	Polyvinylidene Fluoride	聚偏氟乙烯
CCK-8	Cell Counting Kit-8	细胞计数法
SCID	Severe Combined Immunodeficiency	重症联合免疫缺陷
IACUC	Institutional Animal Care and Use Committee	动物保护与利用委员会
ICP-MS	Inductively Coupled Plasma Mass Spectrometry	电感耦合等离子体质谱
H-E	Hematoxylin and Eosin	苏木精-伊红
WBC	White Blood Cell	白细胞
NEU	Neutrophil	中性粒细胞
LYM	Lymphocyte	淋巴细胞
RBC	Red Blood Cell	红细胞
HGB	Hemoglobin	血红蛋白
PLT	Platelet	血小板
ALT	Alanine Aminotransferase	谷丙转氨酶
AST	Aspartate Aminotransferase	谷草转氨酶
BUN	Blood Urea Nitrogen	血尿素氮

续表

英文缩写	英文全称	中文全称
Scr	Serum creatinine	血肌酐
SD	Standard Deviation	标准差
EPR	Enhanced Permeability and Retention	高通透性和滞留
NADH	Nicotinamide Adenine Dinucleotide	烟酰胺腺嘌呤二核苷酸
GAPDH	Glyceraldehyde-3-phosphate Dehydrogenase	甘油醛-3-磷酸脱氢酶
SUV	Standard Uptake Value	标准摄取值
VEGF	Vascular Endothelial Growth Factor	血管内皮生长因子
NRP-1	Neuropilin-1	神经肽-1
HSPs	Heat Shock Proteins	热休克蛋白
Cy5.5	Cyanine 5.5 Amine	菁5.5胺
WCl_6	Tungsten Hexachloride	六氯化钨
PAA	Poly Acrylic Acid	聚丙烯酸
DEG	Diethylene Glycol	二甘醇
EDC	Ethyl Dimethylaminopropyl Carbodiimide	乙基二甲氨基丙基碳化二亚胺
JSPDC	Joint Committee on Powder Diffraction Standards	粉末衍射标准联合委员会

后记

近红外多功能纳米探针的构建及其在胃肠道恶性肿瘤诊断与治疗中的应用

胃肠道恶性肿瘤是严重威胁人类健康的重大疾病,其早期准确诊断和有效治疗对于改善患者预后至关重要。传统的诊断和治疗方法存在诸多局限性,而近红外多功能纳米探针的出现为胃肠道恶性肿瘤的诊疗带来了新的机遇和突破。

1. 近红外多功能纳米探针的构建

(1) 材料选择

近红外多功能纳米探针的构建首先涉及合适材料的选取。常见的材料包括量子点、金纳米粒子、碳纳米管、稀土掺杂纳米材料等。这些材料具有独特的光学、物理和化学性质,使其在近红外区域表现出良好的荧光发射、光热转换等特性。例如,量子点具有尺寸可调的荧光发射波长、高量子产率等优点;金纳米粒子则具备良好的生物相容性、表面易修饰以及独特的局域表面等离子体共振效应,可实现光热治疗等功能。

(2) 功能化修饰

为了赋予纳米探针更多的功能,如靶向性、药物负载等,通常需要对其进行功能化修饰。通过在纳米粒子表面连接特异性的靶向配体,如抗体、多肽、小分子等,可以实现纳米探针对胃肠道恶性肿瘤细胞的特异性识别和结合。例如,将针对胃肠道肿瘤相关抗原的抗体修饰在纳米探针表面,使其能够精准地定位到肿瘤细胞。同时,还可以利用纳米粒子的多孔结构或表面化学键合等方式负载化疗药物、基因药物等,实现诊断与治疗一体化的功能。

(3) 合成方法

多种合成方法被用于构建近红外多功能纳米探针。例如,化学共沉淀法可用于合成量子点等纳米材料,种子生长法常用于制备金纳米粒子,水热合成法在一些复杂结构的纳米材料合成中发挥重要作用。这些合成方法各有优劣,需要根据具体的材料和功能要求进行选择和优化,以确保合成出的纳米探针具有良好的均一性、稳定性和所需的性能。

2. 在胃肠道恶性肿瘤诊断中的应用

(1) 荧光成像诊断

近红外多功能纳米探针的荧光成像功能是其在诊断中的重要应用之一。由于近红外光在生物组织中的穿透深度相对较大,且组织自发荧光干扰较小,纳米探针发出的近红外荧光可以清晰地显示胃肠道恶性肿瘤的位置、大小和形态。通过静脉注射或口服等给药方式,纳米探针能够在体内循环并特异性地聚集在肿瘤部位,然后利用荧光成像设备,如荧光显微镜、小动物活体成像仪等进行实时监测和成像。这种成像方式不仅可以用于肿瘤的早期筛查,还可以在手术过程中辅助确定肿瘤边界,提高手术切除的准确性。

(2) 光声成像诊断

除了荧光成像,光声成像也是近红外多功能纳米探针的重要诊断应用。光声成像结合了光学成像的高对比度和超声成像的高穿透深度的优点。当纳米探针吸收近红外激光脉冲后,会产生光热效应并引起周围组织的热膨胀,从而产生超声波信号。通过检测这些超声波信号并进行成像处理,可以获得胃肠道恶性肿瘤的清晰图像。光声成像对于深层肿瘤的检测以及对肿瘤血管分布等情况的评估具有独特的优势,能够为肿瘤的诊断和治疗方案的制定提供更全面的信息。

(3) 多模态成像诊断

为了进一步提高诊断的准确性和全面性,近红外多功能纳米探针还可实现多模态成像诊断。例如,将荧光成像与光声成像相结合,或者再加入磁共振成像(MRI)、计算机断层扫描(CT)等其他成像模态的功能。通过不同成像模态的优势互补,可以从多个角度、多个层面获取胃肠道恶性肿瘤的信息。比如,MRI 可以提供肿瘤组织的精细解剖结构信息,CT 可以清晰显示肿瘤的钙化等情况,再结合纳米探针的近红外荧光成像和光声成像,能够更加准确地判断肿瘤的性质、分期等,为后续的治疗提供更精准的依据。

3. 在胃肠道恶性肿瘤治疗中的应用

(1) 光热治疗

近红外多功能纳米探针的光热转换特性使其可用于胃肠道恶性肿瘤的光热治疗。当纳米探针聚集在肿瘤部位后,通过外部近红外激光照射,纳米探针能够将吸收的光能高效转化为热能,使肿瘤组织局部温度迅速升高。一般当温度达到 42~45 ℃以上时,就可以对肿瘤细胞产生不可逆的损伤,导致细胞凋亡或坏死。光热治疗具有靶向性强、副作用相对较小等优点,而且可以与其他治疗方法如化疗、放疗等联合使用,提高治疗效果。

(2) 化疗协同治疗

如前文所述,纳米探针可以负载化疗药物。在治疗过程中,一方面纳米探针通过靶向作用将化疗药物精准地输送到肿瘤部位,减少药物对正常组织的毒副作用;另一方面,光热治疗所产生的局部高温环境可以增强化疗药物的疗效。

例如,高温可以促进肿瘤细胞对化疗药物的摄取,破坏肿瘤细胞的耐药机制等,从而实现光热治疗与化疗的协同作用,更有效地杀灭肿瘤细胞。

(3) 基因治疗协同治疗

除了化疗,近红外多功能纳米探针还可与基因治疗协同,可以将基因药物如小干扰 RNA(siRNA)、质粒 DNA 等负载到纳米探针上,通过靶向输送到肿瘤细胞内。光热治疗产生的局部高温同样可以促进基因药物进入细胞并发挥作用,比如提高基因转染效率等。同时,基因治疗可以从根本上纠正肿瘤细胞的异常基因表达,与光热治疗等物理治疗方法相结合,有望为胃肠道恶性肿瘤的治疗提供新的思路和更有效的治疗方案。

4. 面临的挑战与解决策略

(1) 体内稳定性

近红外多功能纳米探针在体内可能会面临稳定性不足的问题,如纳米粒子的团聚、降解等,这会影响其诊断和治疗效果。解决策略包括优化纳米探针的合成工艺,提高其自身的稳定性;通过表面修饰等方式增加纳米粒子与生物环境的相容性,减少与生物分子的相互作用导致的不稳定因素。

(2) 生物安全性

纳米探针进入人体后,其生物安全性是需要重点关注的问题。虽然目前所选用的许多材料具有一定的生物相容性,但长期的生物效应仍需进一步研究。需要开展更多的体内外生物安全性评估实验,如细胞毒性测试、动物长期毒性观察等,并且根据评估结果对纳米探针的设计和材料选择进行优化,确保其在应用过程中不会对人体造成潜在的危害。

(3) 临床转化

将近红外多功能纳米探针从实验室研究成果转化为临床应用还面临诸多困难。包括临床试验的设计和开展难度较大,需要满足严格的伦理要求和监管标准;成本问题也是一个重要因素,目前构建和生产纳米探针的成本相对较高,不利于其大规模临床推广。解决这些问题需要加强产学研合作,整合各方资源,推动纳米探针的临床前研究向临床应用的顺利过渡。

5. 总结

近红外多功能纳米探针的构建为胃肠道恶性肿瘤的诊断与治疗带来了诸多优势和新的可能性。通过合理选择材料、进行功能化修饰和优化合成方法,可以构建出具有良好性能的纳米探针,实现其在荧光成像、光声成像、多模态成像等方面的诊断功能,以及光热治疗、化疗协同、基因治疗协同等治疗功能。然而,在其发展过程中也面临着体内稳定性、生物安全性和临床转化等诸多挑战。未来,需要进一步深入研究,不断优化纳米探针的设计和性能,加强生物安全性评估,推动临床转化工作,以便使近红外多功能纳米探针能够真正广泛应用于胃肠道恶性肿瘤的临床诊疗,为改善患者的健康状况和提高患者的生活质量做出更大的贡献。